THE ESSENCIAL ALKALINE DIET COOKBOOK FOR BEGINNERS

I0146437

100+ Alkaline Recipes to Bring Your Body Back to Balance! Healthy Recipes to Enjoy Favorite Foods for Weight-Loss!

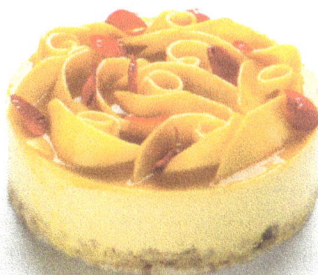

By

Laura Green

TABLE OF CONTENT

INTRODUCTION

It is essential to support the alkalinity of the body by maintaining the suitable pH of the blood. In addition, it helps maintain the health of your body by keeping you away from ailments that include kidney stones, heart disease, and cancer. One of the best ways to achieve alkaline-acid balance is to follow the alkaline diet.

The diet helps you lose weight, but it has more health benefits besides keeping you fit. Like any type of diet, not everyone finds it easy, especially since most of the foods you'll be eating are fruits and vegetables.

This cookbook is a handy companion for people who want to benefit from the diet without quickly getting tired of eating almost the same ingredients over and over again. In addition to explaining everything you need to know about alkaline and acid and how they affect your blood pH, it contains many helpful tips to make the transition more accessible and enjoyable.

WHY AN ALKALINE DIET?

The diet focus is a philosophy that believes that the foods we eat can easily alter our body chemistry. It all depends on whether the food is alkaline or acidic. Our body's pH will change depending on the foods we eat.

You have to understand that when your body needs energy, it starts burning food. This process is very controlled and takes place in an environment that our body controls. When our body absorbed the foods we consume and gets energy from them, we burn the foods but in a very controlled and slow manner. This is what is known as metabolism, the conversion of food into energy. This works a lot like a fire because it involves a chemical reaction to break down the food. These chemical reactions happen in a controlled and slow manner.

It is just like when we burn wood in the oven; when we burn food, it produces waste that is sometimes called "ash." This waste product can be either alkaline or acidic.

These "ashes" are what alters the pH of our bodies. It all depends on the mineral, sulfur, or protein content of the food. Consuming foods that leave acidic ash such as refined carbohydrates, processed foods, fried foods, or sugar can, over time, increase inflammation, and this leaves us vulnerable to disease. Although our bodies are exposed to vast amounts of acidic "ash," they will slowly become more susceptible to disease because the immune system is weakening.

Our bodies house many organs that are very good at eliminating and neutralizing acid. Our bodies can resist up to a certain acidic pH. The alkaline diet does not attempt to change the pH of the blood, but it removes the stress of trying to maintain a healthy pH in the body by giving it the tools to thrive. Foods that are formed alkaline, such as plant proteins, tubers, vegetables, and whole fruits, are all alkaline because they are anti-inflammatory, natural, fresh, delicious foods rich in antioxidants, chlorophyll, minerals, and vitamins. On the other hand, when our bloodstream is affected by a significant alkalinity level, it forms a protective layer that will keep our body healthy.

This diet is more of an eating plan than a diet. It is used to improve our health. Because it emphasizes fresh fruits and vegetables, it is based on the idea that after the foods we eat are absorbed and digested; they reach the kidneys as eight compounds that form bases or acids.

There have been many techniques used to look at foods and figure out their base or acid load in the body. Some foods will be more basic or acidic than others. Surprisingly, cheddar is more acidic than egg whites. Spinach is more basic than watermelon.

It is thought that a diet high in acidic foods disrupts the pH level of the blood and triggers the loss of minerals such as calcium as the body tries to restore its natural balance. This imbalance is what makes us susceptible to disease.

The alkaline diet not only helps improve your health, but it can slow down the aging process, preserve muscle mass and protect against many other health problems such as osteoporosis, kidney stones, cardiovascular disease, diabetes, and the common cold. This diet can also help you lose weight and increase your energy levels.

For these reasons, it is recommended that you try to choose foods that are high in alkalinity.

The following classifies the various types of foods according to their "ash."

- Alkaline: Foods such as fruits, nuts, legumes, and vegetables.
- Neutral: Foods containing starches, fats, and sugars
- Acidic: Foods such as alcohol, eggs, grains, dairy products, poultry, fish, and meat

Here's some background on the alkalinity/acidity of a regular diet and points about how this diet can help the human body:

- Researchers think there has been a considerable change from the starvation/gathering civilization to the one we have today. With the agricultural revolution and the mass industrialization of the foods we eat over the last 200 years, the foods we eat have much less chloride, magnesium, and potassium. They have much more sodium than other diets.

- Our kidneys maintain normal electrolyte levels. When the kidneys are exposed to very acidic substances, electrolytes must be used to combat the acidity.

- The ratio of sodium to potassium in regular diets today has changed dramatically. Potassium should outnumber sodium ten to one, but the ratio has dropped to one to three. So, when we eat a "normal" American diet, we now eat three times as much sodium as potassium on an average day.

- These changes in our diet have caused an increase in metabolic acidosis. This means that the pH levels in our bodies are no longer optimal. In addition to this, most people suffer from problems such as magnesium and potassium deficiency.

- This causes acceleration of the aging process, degeneration of bone mass and tissues, and gradual loss of organ function. In addition, due to the high degree of acidity in our body, this forces our body to get the minerals it needs from our tissues, organs, cells, and bones.

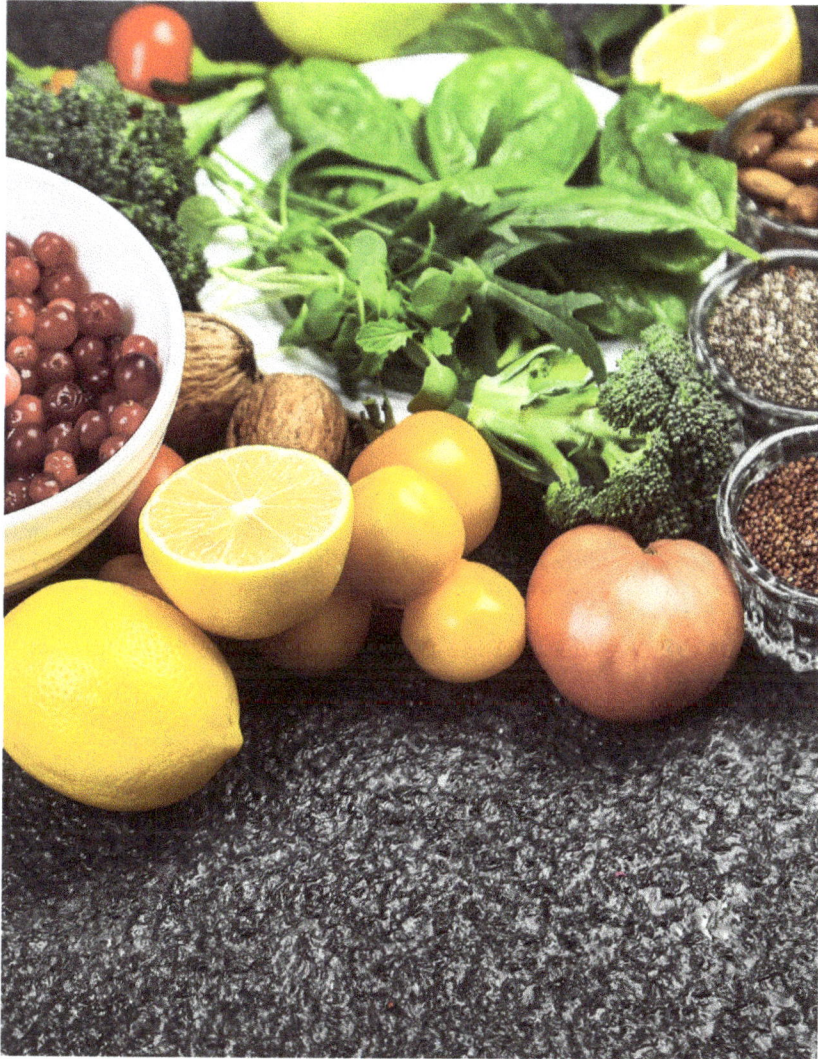

1) Raspberry and banana smoothie bowl

Preparation time: 10 minutes   **Cooking time:** 10 minutes   **Portions: 2**

Ingredients:

- ✓ 2 cups of fresh raspberries, split
- ✓ 2 large frozen bananas, peeled

Ingredients:

- ✓ ½ cup unsweetened almond milk
- ✓ 1/3 cup of fresh mixed berries

Directions:

- ❖ In a blender, add the raspberries, bananas and almond milk and blend until smooth.

- ❖ Transfer the smoothie evenly into two serving bowls.
- ❖ Top each bowl with berries and serve immediately.

2) Apple and walnut porridge

Preparation time: 10 minutes   **Cooking time:** 5 minutes   **Portions: 4**

Ingredients:

- ✓ 2 cups unsweetened almond milk
- ✓ 3 tablespoons walnuts, chopped
- ✓ 3 tablespoons of sunflower seeds
- ✓ 2 large apples, peeled, stoned and grated

Ingredients:

- ✓ ½ teaspoon organic vanilla extract
- ✓ Pinch of cinnamon powder
- ✓ ½ small apple, core and slices
- ✓ 1 small banana, peeled and sliced
- ❖ Remove from the heat and transfer the oatmeal to serving bowls.
- ❖ Cover with apple and banana slices and serve.

Directions:

- ❖ In a large pan, mix together the milk, walnuts, sunflower seeds, applesauce, vanilla and cinnamon over medium-low heat and cook for about 3-5 minutes, stirring often.

3) Chia seed pudding

Preparation time: 10 minutes   **Cooking time:** 10 minutes   **Portions: 3**

Ingredients:

- ✓ 2 cups unsweetened almond milk
- ✓ ½ cup chia seeds
- ✓ 1 tablespoon maple syrup

Ingredients:

- ✓ 1 teaspoon organic vanilla extract
- ✓ 1/3 cup fresh strawberries, hulled and sliced
- ✓ 2 tablespoons of sliced almonds

- ❖ Cover the bowl and refrigerate for at least 3-4 hours, stirring occasionally.
- ❖ Serve with a garnish of strawberries and almonds.

Directions:

- ❖ In a large bowl, add the almond milk, chia seeds, maple syrup and vanilla extract and stir to combine well.

4) Banana and almond smoothie

Preparation time: 10 minutes   **Cooking time:** 0 minutes   **Portions: 2**

Ingredients:

- ✓ 2 large frozen bananas, peeled and sliced
- ✓ 1 tablespoon chopped almonds

Ingredients:

- ✓ 1 teaspoon organic vanilla extract
- ✓ 2 cups of cooled unsweetened almond milk

- ❖ Pour the smoothie into two serving glasses and serve immediately.

Directions:

- ❖ Place all ingredients in a high-speed blender and pulse until smooth and creamy.

5) Strawberry and beetroot smoothie

Preparation time: 10 minutes   **Cooking time**: 0 minutes   **Portions: 2**

Ingredients:

- ✓   2 cups frozen strawberries, hulled
- ✓   2/3 cup frozen beetroot, cut, peeled and chopped
- ✓   1 teaspoon fresh ginger root, peeled and grated

Directions:

- ❖   Place all ingredients in a high-speed blender and pulse until smooth and creamy.

Ingredients:

- ✓   1 teaspoon fresh turmeric root, peeled and grated
- ✓   ½ cup of fresh orange juice
- ✓   1 cup unsweetened almond milk
- ❖   Pour the smoothie into two serving glasses and serve immediately.

6) Raspberry and tofu smoothie

Preparation time: 10 minutes   **Cooking time:**   **Portions: 2**

Ingredients:

- ✓   1½ cups of fresh raspberries
- ✓   6 ounces of firm, drained, pressed and chopped silken tofu
- ✓   1 teaspoon stevia powder

Directions:

- ❖   Place all ingredients in a high-speed blender and pulse until smooth and creamy.

Ingredients:

- ✓   1/8 teaspoon organic vanilla extract
- ✓   1½ cups unsweetened almond milk
- ✓   ¼ cup ice cubes, crushed
- ❖   Pour the smoothie into two serving glasses and serve immediately.

7) Mango and lemon smoothie

Preparation time: 10 minutes   **Cooking time:**   **Portions: 2**

Ingredients:

- ✓   2 cups frozen mango, peeled, stoned and chopped
- ✓   ¼ cup almond butter
- ✓   pinch of ground turmeric

Directions:

- ❖   Place all ingredients in a high-speed blender and pulse until smooth and creamy.

Ingredients:

- ✓   2 tablespoons fresh lemon juice
- ✓   1¼ cup unsweetened almond milk
- ✓   ¼ cup ice cubes, crushed
- ❖   Pour the smoothie into two serving glasses and serve immediately.

8) Papaya and banana smoothie

Preparation time: 10 minutes   **Cooking time:**   **Portions: 2**

Ingredients:

- ✓   ½ of a medium-sized papaya, peeled and roughly chopped
- ✓   1 large banana, peeled and sliced
- ✓   2 tablespoons agave nectar
- ✓   ¼ teaspoon ground turmeric

Directions:

- ❖   Place all ingredients in a high-speed blender and pulse until smooth and creamy.

Ingredients:

- ✓   1 tablespoon fresh lime juice
- ✓   1½ cups unsweetened almond milk
- ✓   ½ cup ice cubes, crushed
- ❖   Pour the smoothie into two serving glasses and serve immediately.

9) Orange and oat smoothie

Preparation time: 10 minutes   **Cooking time**:   **Portions: 2**

Ingredients:
- ✓ 2/3 cups rolled oats
- ✓ 2 oranges, peeled, seeded and cut into pieces
- ✓ 2 large bananas, peeled and sliced

Directions:
- ❖ Place all ingredients in a high-speed blender and pulse until smooth and creamy.

Ingredients:
- ✓ 1½ cups unsweetened almond milk
- ✓ ½ cup ice cubes, crushed

❖ Pour the smoothie into two serving glasses and serve immediately.

10) Pineapple and kale smoothie

Preparation time: 10 minutes   **Cooking time**:   **Portions: 2**

Ingredients:
- ✓ 1½ cups fresh cabbage, hard ribs removed and chopped
- ✓ 1 large frozen banana, peeled and sliced
- ✓ ½ cup of fresh pineapple, peeled and cut into pieces

Directions:
- ❖ Place all ingredients in a high-speed blender and pulse until smooth and creamy.

Ingredients:
- ✓ ½ cup of fresh orange juice
- ✓ 1 cup unsweetened coconut milk
- ✓ ½ cup ice cubes, crushed

❖ Pour the smoothie into two serving glasses and serve immediately.

11) Pumpkin and banana smoothie

Preparation time: 10 minutes   **Cooking time**:   **Portions: 2**

Ingredients:
- ✓ 1 cup of homemade pumpkin puree
- ✓ 1 large banana, peeled and sliced
- ✓ 1 tablespoon maple syrup
- ✓ 1 teaspoon ground linseed

Directions:
- ❖ Place all ingredients in a high-speed blender and pulse until smooth and creamy.

Ingredients:
- ✓ ¼ teaspoon cinnamon powder
- ✓ 1/8 teaspoon ground ginger
- ✓ 1½ cups unsweetened almond milk
- ✓ ¼ cup ice cubes, crushed

❖ Pour the smoothie into two serving glasses and serve immediately.

12) Cabbage and avocado smoothie

Preparation time: 10 minutes   **Cooking time**:   **Portions: 2**

Ingredients:
- ✓ 2 cups fresh cabbage, hard ribs removed and chopped
- ✓ ½ of a medium avocado, peeled, pitted and chopped
- ✓ ½ inch pieces of fresh ginger root, peeled and chopped

Directions:
- ❖ Place all ingredients in a high-speed blender and pulse until smooth and creamy.

Ingredients:
- ✓ ½ inch pieces of fresh turmeric root, peeled and chopped
- ✓ 1½ cups unsweetened coconut milk
- ✓ ¼ cup ice cubes, crushed

❖ Pour the smoothie into two serving glasses and serve immediately.

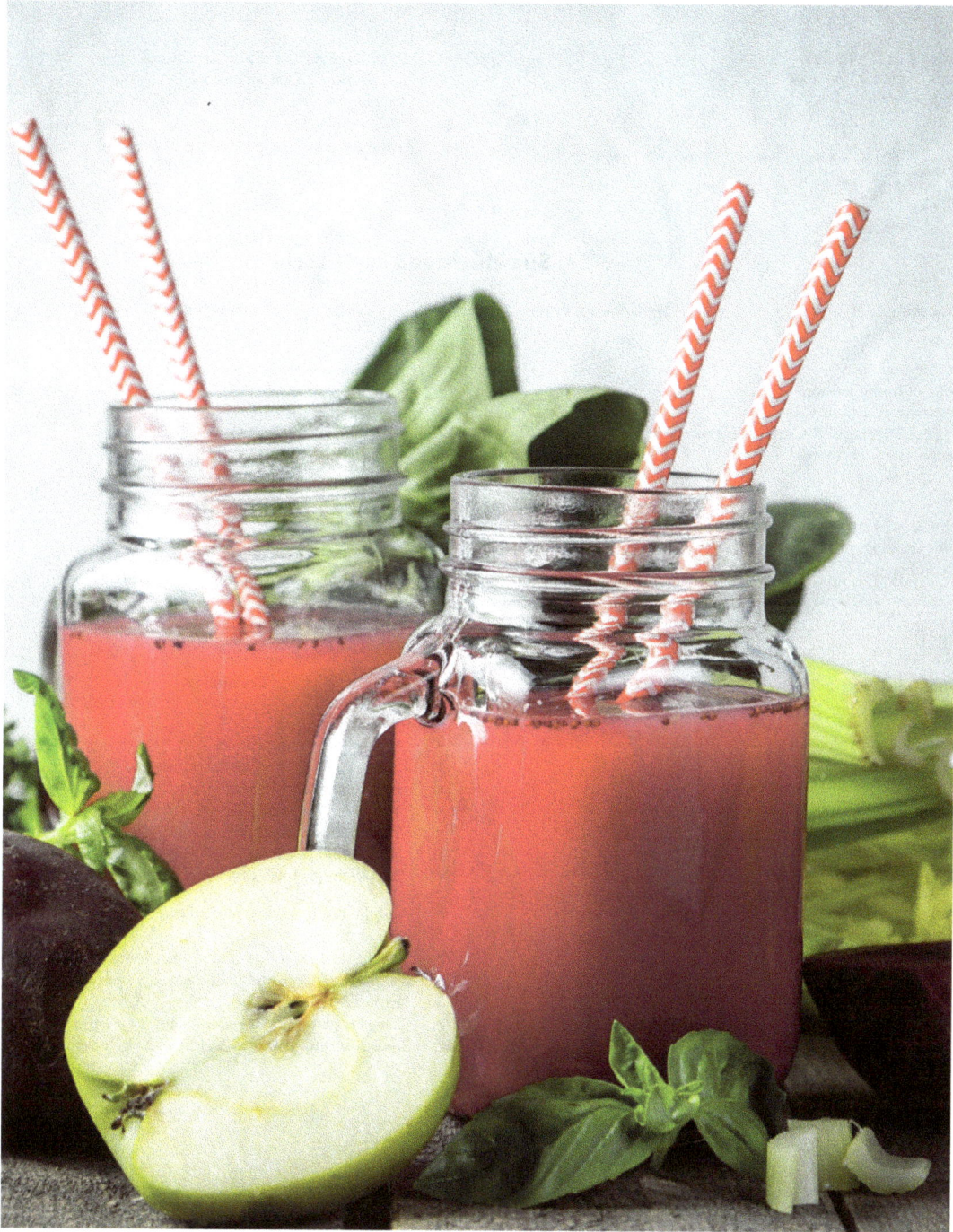

13) Tomato and vegetable salad

Preparation time: 15 minutes.   **Cooking time**:   **Portions: 4**

Ingredients:
- ✓ 6 cups of fresh vegetables
- ✓ 2 cups of cherry tomatoes
- ✓ 2 shallots, chopped

Directions:
- ❖ Place all the ingredients in a large bowl and mix to coat well.

Ingredients:
- ✓ 2 tablespoons of extra virgin olive oil
- ✓ 2 tablespoons fresh orange juice
- ✓ 1 tablespoon fresh lemon juice
- ❖ Cover the bowl and refrigerate for about 6-8 hours.
- ❖ Remove from the fridge and stir well before serving.

14) Strawberry and apple salad

Preparation time: 15 minutes.   **Cooking time**:   **Portions: 4**

Ingredients:
- For the salad:
- ✓ 4 cups of mixed lettuce, torn up
- ✓ 2 apples, core and slices
- ✓ 1 cup fresh strawberries, peeled and sliced
- ✓ ¼ cup pecans, chopped
- For the dressing:

Directions:
- ❖ For the salad, place all the ingredients in a large bowl and mix well.
- ❖ For the dressing, place all the ingredients in a bowl and whisk until well combined.

Ingredients:
- ✓ 3 tablespoons apple cider vinegar
- ✓ 3 tablespoons of olive oil
- ✓ 1 tablespoon agave nectar
- ✓ 1 teaspoon poppy seeds

- ❖ Pour the dressing over the salad and toss to coat well.
- ❖ Serve immediately.

15) Cauliflower soup

Preparation time: 15 minutes   **Cooking time:** 30 minutes.   **Portions: 4**

Ingredients:
- ✓ 2 tablespoons of olive oil
- ✓ 1 yellow onion, chopped
- ✓ 2 carrots, peeled and cut into pieces
- ✓ 2 cloves of garlic, minced
- ✓ 1 Serrano pepper, finely chopped
- ✓ 2 stalks of celery, chopped
- ✓ 1 teaspoon ground turmeric
- ✓ 1 teaspoon ground coriander

Directions:
- ❖ Heat the oil over a medium heat in a large soup pot and fry the onion, carrot and celery for about 4-6 minutes.
- ❖ Add the garlic, serrano pepper and spices and fry for about 1 minute.
- ❖ Add the cauliflower and cook for about 5 minutes, stirring occasionally.

Ingredients:
- ✓ 1 teaspoon ground cumin
- ✓ ¼ teaspoon red pepper flakes, crushed
- ✓ 1 head of cauliflower, chopped
- ✓ 4 cups of homemade vegetable stock
- ✓ 1 cup unsweetened coconut milk
- ✓ Sea salt and freshly ground black pepper, to taste
- ✓ 2 tablespoons fresh chives, finely chopped

- ❖ Add the broth and coconut milk and bring to the boil over medium-high heat.
- ❖ Reduce the heat to low and simmer for about 15 minutes.
- ❖ Season the soup with salt and black pepper and remove from the heat.
- ❖ Using an immersion blender, blend the soup until smooth.
- ❖ Serve hot and garnish with chives.

16) Tomato soup

Preparation time: 15 minutes   **Cooking time:** 45 minutes   **Portions: 4**

Ingredients:

- ✓ 2 tablespoons of coconut oil
- ✓ 2 carrots, coarsely chopped
- ✓ 1 large white onion, coarsely chopped
- ✓ 3 cloves of garlic, minced
- ✓ 5 large tomatoes, roughly chopped

Directions:

- ❖ Melt the coconut oil in a large soup pot over medium heat and cook the carrot and onion for about 10 minutes, stirring often.
- ❖ Add the garlic and fry for about 1-2 minutes.
- ❖ Add the tomatoes, tomato paste, basil, stock, salt and black pepper and bring to the boil.

Ingredients:

- ✓ 1 tablespoon homemade tomato paste
- ✓ 3 cups of homemade vegetable stock
- ✓ ¼ cup fresh basil, chopped
- ✓ ¼ cup unsweetened coconut milk
- ✓ Sea salt and freshly ground black pepper, to taste
- ❖ Reduce the heat to low and simmer uncovered for about 30 minutes.
- ❖ Add the coconut milk and remove from the heat.
- ❖ Using an immersion blender, blend the soup until smooth.
- ❖ Serve hot.

17) Garlic broccoli

Preparation time: 10 minutes   **Cooking time:** 8 minutes   **Portions: 2**

Ingredients:

- ✓ 1 tablespoon extra virgin olive oil
- ✓ 3-4 garlic cloves, minced

Directions:

- ❖ Heat the oil over medium heat in a large frying pan and fry the garlic for about 1 minute.
- ❖ Add the broccoli and fry for about 2 minutes.

Ingredients:

- ✓ 2 cups of broccoli florets
- ✓ 2 tablespoons of tamari
- ❖ Add the tamari and stir-fry for about 4-5 minutes or until cooked through.
- ❖ Remove from the heat and serve hot.

18) Gombo al curry

Preparation time: 10 minutes   **Cooking time:** 15 minutes   **Portions: 3**

Ingredients:

- ✓ 1 tablespoon olive oil
- ✓ ½ teaspoon of caraway seeds
- ✓ ¾ lb okra pods, trimmed and cut into 2 inch pieces
- ✓ ½ teaspoon of curry powder

Directions:

- ❖ Heat the oil in a large frying pan over medium heat.
- ❖ For about 30 seconds, sauté the cumin seeds
- ❖ Add the okra and fry for about 1-1½ minutes.
- ❖ Reduce the heat to low and cook covered for about 6-8 minutes, stirring occasionally.

Ingredients:

- ✓ ½ teaspoon of red chilli powder
- ✓ 1 teaspoon ground coriander
- ✓ Sea salt and freshly ground black pepper, to taste

- ❖ Add the curry powder, red pepper and cilantro and stir to combine.
- ❖ Increase the heat to medium and cook uncovered for a further 2-3 minutes or so.
- ❖ Season with salt and pepper and remove from the heat.
- ❖ Serve hot.

19) Mushroom curry

Preparation time: 20 minutes   **Cooking time:** 20 minutes   **Portions: 4**

Ingredients:
- ✓ 2 cups of tomatoes, chopped
- ✓ 1 green chilli, chopped
- ✓ 1 teaspoon fresh ginger, chopped
- ✓ 2 tablespoons of olive oil
- ✓ ½ teaspoon of caraway seeds
- ✓ ¼ teaspoon of ground coriander
- ✓ ¼ teaspoon ground turmeric

Directions:
- ❖ In a food processor, add the tomatoes, green chillies and ginger and pulse until a smooth paste is formed.
- ❖ Heat the oil in a frying pan over medium heat.
- ❖ For about 1 minute, fry the cumin seeds.
- ❖ Add the spices and fry for about 1 minute.

Ingredients:
- ✓ ¼ teaspoon of red chilli powder
- ✓ 2 cups fresh shiitake mushrooms, sliced
- ✓ 2 cups fresh button mushrooms, sliced
- ✓ 1¼ cup water
- ✓ ¼ cup unsweetened coconut milk
- ✓ Sea salt and freshly ground black pepper, to taste

- ❖ Add the tomato mixture and cook for about 5 minutes.
- ❖ Add the mushrooms, water and coconut milk and bring to the boil.
- ❖ Cook for about 10-12 minutes, stirring occasionally.
- ❖ Season with salt and black pepper and remove from the heat.
- ❖ Serve hot.

20) Glazed Brussels sprouts

Preparation time: 15 minutes   **Cooking time:** 15 minutes   **Portions: 3**

Ingredients:
- ✓ 3 cups Brussels sprouts, cut and halved
- ✓ Sea salt, to taste
- ✓ 2 tablespoons coconut oil, melted
- ✓ For the orange glaze:
- ✓ 1 tablespoon of coconut oil
- ✓ 2 small shallots, thinly sliced

Directions:
- ❖ Preheat the oven to 400 degrees F. Line a baking tray with baking paper.
- ❖ In a bowl, add the Brussels sprouts, a little salt and oil and stir to coat well.
- ❖ Transfer the mixture into the prepared baking tin.
- ❖ Roast for about 10-15 minutes, turning once halfway through.
- ❖ Meanwhile, prepare the icing.
- ❖ In a frying pan, melt the coconut oil over medium heat and fry the shallots for about 5 minutes.
- ❖ Add the orange zest and fry for about 1 minute.

Ingredients:
- ✓ 2 tablespoons fresh orange zest, finely grated
- ✓ ¼ teaspoon of ground ginger
- ✓ 2/3 cup fresh orange juice
- ✓ 1 tablespoon sambal oelek (raw chilli paste)
- ✓ 2 tablespoons of coconut amino acids
- ✓ 1 teaspoon tapioca starch
- ✓ Sea salt, to taste
- ❖ Stir in the ginger, orange juice, sambal oelek and coconut amino acid and cook for about 5 minutes.
- ❖ Slowly add the tapioca starch, whisking constantly.
- ❖ Cook for a further 2-3 minutes, stirring frequently.
- ❖ Add salt and remove from the heat.
- ❖ Transfer the roasted Brussels sprouts to a serving dish. Top evenly with the orange glaze.
- ❖ Serve immediately garnished with shallots.

21) Sautéed mushrooms

Preparation time: 15 minutes   **Cooking time:** 16 minutes   **Portions: 2**

Ingredients:
- ✓ 2 tablespoons of olive oil
- ✓ ½ teaspoon caraway seeds, slightly crushed
- ✓ 2 medium onions, thinly sliced

Directions:
- ❖ Heat oil in a frying pan over medium heat.
- ❖ For about 1 minute, fry the cumin seeds.
- ❖ Add the onion and fry for about 4-5 minutes.

Ingredients:
- ✓ ¾ lb fresh mushrooms, chopped
- ✓ Sea salt and freshly ground black pepper, to taste

- ❖ Add the mushrooms and fry for about 5-7 minutes.
- ❖ Add salt and black pepper and fry for about 2-3 minutes.
- ❖ Remove from the heat and serve hot.

22) Sweet and sour cabbage

Preparation time: 10 minutes   **Cooking time:** 20 minutes   **Portions: 4**

Ingredients:

- ✓ 1 tablespoon extra virgin olive oil
- ✓ 1 lemon, seeded and thinly sliced
- ✓ 1 onion, chopped
- ✓ 3 cloves of garlic, minced

Directions:

- ❖ In a large frying pan, heat the oil over medium heat and cook the lemon slices for about 5 minutes.
- ❖ Using a slotted spoon, remove the lemon slices.

Ingredients:

- ✓ 2 lbs. fresh cabbage, hard ribs removed and chopped
- ✓ ½ cup shallots, chopped
- ✓ 1 tablespoon agave nectar
- ✓ Sea salt and freshly ground black pepper, to taste
- ❖ In the same pan, add the onion and garlic and fry for about 5 minutes.
- ❖ Add the cabbage, shallots, agave nectar, salt and black pepper and cook for about 8-10 minutes, stirring occasionally.
- ❖ Remove from the heat and serve hot.

23) Brussels sprouts with walnuts

Preparation time: 15 minutes   **Cooking time:** 15 minutes   **Portions: 2**

Ingredients:

- ✓ ½ pound Brussels sprouts, halved
- ✓ 1 tablespoon olive oil
- ✓ 2 cloves of garlic, minced
- ✓ ½ teaspoon red pepper flakes, crushed

Directions:

- ❖ Place a steamer basket in a large pot of boiling water.
- ❖ Place the Brussels sprouts in the basket of the steamer and steam, covered, for about 6-8 minutes.
- ❖ Drain the Brussels sprouts well.
- ❖ In a large frying pan, heat the oil over medium heat and fry the garlic and red pepper flakes for about 40 seconds.

Ingredients:

- ✓ Sea salt and freshly ground black pepper, to taste
- ✓ 1 tablespoon fresh lemon juice
- ✓ 1 tablespoon pine nuts

- ❖ Add the Brussels sprouts, salt and black pepper and fry for about 4-5 minutes.
- ❖ Add the lemon juice and fry for about 1 minute more.
- ❖ Add the pine nuts and remove from the heat.
- ❖ Serve hot.

24) Roasted pumpkin by Butternut

Preparation time: 15 minutes   **Cooking time:** 45 minutes   **Portions: 6**

Ingredients:

- ✓ 8 cups butternut squash, peeled, seeded and diced
- ✓ 2 tablespoons of melted almond butter
- ✓ ½ teaspoon ground cinnamon

Directions:

- ❖ Preheat the oven to 425 degrees F. Place the pieces of foil on 2 baking sheets.
- ❖ In a large bowl, add all the ingredients and mix to coat well.

Ingredients:

- ✓ ½ teaspoon ground cumin
- ✓ ¼ teaspoon red pepper flakes
- ✓ Sea salt, to taste
- ❖ Arrange the pumpkin pieces on the prepared baking trays in a single layer.
- ❖ Roast for about 40-45 minutes.
- ❖ Remove from the oven and serve.

25) Broccoli with peppers

Preparation time: 15 minutes   **Cooking time:** 10 minutes   **Portions: 4**

Ingredients:

- ✓ 2 tablespoons of olive oil
- ✓ 4 cloves of garlic, minced
- ✓ 1 large white onion, sliced
- ✓ 2 cups of small broccoli florets

Directions:

- ❖ In a large frying pan, heat the oil over medium heat and fry the garlic for about 1 minute.

Ingredients:

- ✓ 3 red peppers, seeded and sliced
- ✓ ¼ cup of homemade vegetable stock
- ✓ Sea salt and freshly ground black pepper, to taste

- ❖ Add the onion, broccoli and peppers and fry for about 5 minutes.
- ❖ Add the stock and fry for about 4 minutes more.
- ❖ Serve hot.

26) Prawns with tamari

Preparation time: 15 minutes   **Cooking time:** 6 minutes   **Portions: 2**

Ingredients:
- ✓ 1 tablespoon olive oil
- ✓ 2 cloves of garlic, minced
- ✓ ½ pound of raw, peeled and deveined jumbo prawns

Directions:
- ❖ In a large frying pan, heat the oil over medium heat and fry the garlic for about 1 minute.

Ingredients:
- ✓ 2 tablespoons of tamari
- ✓ Freshly ground black pepper, to taste

- ❖ Stir in the prawns, tamari and black pepper and cook for about 4-5 minutes or until fully cooked.
- ❖ Serve hot.

27) Vegetarian kebab

Preparation time: 20 minutes   **Cooking time:** 10 minutes   **Portions: 4**

Ingredients:
  For the marinade:
- ✓ 2 cloves of garlic, minced
- ✓ 2 teaspoons fresh basil, chopped
- ✓ 2 teaspoons fresh oregano, chopped
- ✓ ½ teaspoon of cayenne pepper
- ✓ Sea salt and freshly ground black pepper, to taste
- ✓ 2 tablespoons fresh lemon juice

Directions:
- ❖ For the marinade: in a large bowl, add all the ingredients and mix until well combined.
- ❖ Add the vegetables to the marinade and toss to coat them well.
- ❖ Cover and refrigerate the vegetables to marinate for at least 6-8 hours.
- ❖ In a large bowl of water, soak the wooden skewers for at least 30 minutes.

Ingredients:
- ✓ 2 tablespoons of olive oil
  For the vegetables:
- ✓ 2 large courgettes, cut into thick slices
- ✓ 8 large button mushrooms, quartered
- ✓ 1 yellow pepper, seeded and diced
- ✓ 1 red pepper, seeded and diced

- ❖ Preheat the grill to medium-high heat. Generously grease the grill grate.
- ❖ Remove the vegetables from the bowl and discard the marinade.
- ❖ Thread the vegetables onto the pre-soaked wooden skewers, starting with the courgettes, mushrooms and peppers.
- ❖ Grill for about 8-10 minutes or until cooked through, turning occasionally.

28) Fried onion sprout

Preparation time: 5 minutes   **Cooking time:** 10 minutes   **Portions: 4**

Ingredients:
- ✓ 2½ pounds of Brussels sprouts, cut4 slices of bacon, cut into 1-inch pieces
- ✓ 1 tablespoon extra virgin coconut oil
- ✓ 1 tomato, chopped
- ✓ 1 onion, chopped

Directions:
- ❖ Add the sprouts to boiling water in a pot.
- ❖ Let them cook for about 3-5 minutes.
- ❖ Drain and set aside.
- ❖ Saute the onions in a greased pan for 4 minutes.

Ingredients:
- ✓ 4 sprigs of thyme or savory, split
- ✓ 1 teaspoon Celtic sea salt, iodine-free
- ✓ Freshly ground pepper to taste
- ✓ 2 teaspoons of lemon juice (optional)

- ❖ Mix with salt, pepper and thyme
- ❖ Add the drained sprouts to the pan and stir for 3 minutes.
- ❖ Remove and discard sprigs of herbs.
- ❖ Serve hot with lemon juice and chopped spring onion on top.

29) South West Stuffed Sweet Potatoes

Preparation time: **Cooking time:** **Portions:**

Ingredients:
- ✓ Sliced avocado (1)
- ✓ Pinch of cumin
- ✓ Pinch of dried red chilli flakes
- ✓ Spinach (3 c.)
- ✓ Sliced shallot (1)
- ✓ Black beans (.5 c.)
- ✓ Coconut oil (2 tablespoons)
- ✓ Sweet potatoes

Ingredients:
- ✓ Medicines
- ✓ Pepper and salt
- ✓ Chopped coriander (1 handful)
- ✓ Cumin (1 teaspoon)
- ✓ Lime juice (1)
- ✓ Olive oil (3 tablespoons)

Directions:
- ❖ Turn on the oven and give it time to heat up to 400 degrees. Clean the sweet potatoes and pierce them a few times with a fork.
- ❖ Add baking paper to a baking tray and place the sweet potatoes on it. Add to the oven to bake.
- ❖ After 50 minutes, the potatoes should be soft. Remove them from the oven and give them time to cool.
- ❖ Meanwhile, take a frying pan and add the coconut oil together with the black beans and shallot.

- ❖ Cook these for a few minutes before adding the cumin, chilli flakes and spinach, stirring to mix well.
- ❖ Finally, take a small bowl and whisk well the ingredients for the dressing.
- ❖ Cut the sweet potatoes in half before stuffing them with the black bean mixture you have made.
- ❖ Add a few slices of avocado and some of the dressing poured over it before serving.

30) Zoodles with cream sauce

Preparation time: **Cooking time:** **Portions:**

Ingredients:
- ✓ Toasted pepitas (2 tablespoons)
- ✓ Pepper (.5 tsp.)
- ✓ Salt (1 teaspoon)
- ✓ Chopped coriander (2 tbsp)
- ✓ Water (1 tablespoon)

Ingredients:
- ✓ Lemon juice (.5)
- ✓ Olive oil (2 tablespoons)
- ✓ Pitted avocado (1)
- ✓ Spiral courgettes (1)
- ✓ Coconut oil (1 tablespoon)
- ❖ Add the sauce to the pan with the noodles and stir to combine. Move to a serving bowl and add the rest of the coriander and toasted pepitas before serving.

Directions:
- ❖ Add a little coconut oil to melt in a frying pan before adding the courgette noodles. Cook for 5 minutes before turning off the heat.
- ❖ Take out a blender and combine the pepper, salt, 1 tablespoon of cilantro, water, lemon juice, oil and avocado. Mix well and cook to make the cream.

31) Rainbow Pad Thai

Preparation time: **Cooking time:** **Portions:**

Ingredients:
- ✓ Avocado cubes (1)
- ✓ Chopped coriander (1 c.)
- ✓ Shredded daikon radish (1 c.)
- ✓ Chopped broccoli (1 c.)
- ✓ Shredded red cabbage (1 c.)
- ✓ Sliced shallots (3)
- ✓ Shredded carrots (2)
- ✓ Spiral courgettes (3)

Ingredients:
- For the dressing
- ✓ Chopped ginger (1 teaspoon)
- ✓ Chopped garlic clove (1)
- ✓ Sesame oil (1 tablespoon)
- ✓ Tahini (.25 c.)
- ✓ Lime juice (1)

- ❖ Top the vegetables with the diced avocado and pour the dressing over them before serving.

Directions:
- ❖ Add the ingredients for the Pad Thai, except the avocado, to a large bowl and mix.
- ❖ Blend together all the ingredients you have for the dressing until creamy and combined.

32) Lentils and vegetables

Preparation time:

Cooking time:

Portions:

Ingredients:
- ✓ Avocado (1)
- ✓ Crushed almonds (1 tablespoon)
- ✓ Crushed black pepper (1 teaspoon)
- ✓ Salt (1 teaspoon)
- ✓ Rocket (1c)
- ✓ Brown or green lentils (.5 c.)

Directions:
- ❖ Add the vegetable stock to a pan over medium heat. Let it start to simmer before adding the lemon juice, carrot, broccoli and pak choi.

Ingredients:
- ✓ Cooked wild rice (1 c.)
- ✓ Lemon juice (.5)
- ✓ Diced carrot (1)
- ✓ Broccoli florets (.5 c.)
- ✓ Sliced Pak choi (.5 c.)
- ✓ Vegetable stock (.25 c.)
- ❖ After 5 minutes, turn off the heat and stir in the almonds, pepper, salt, rocket, lentils and wild rice.
- ❖ Place this mixture on plates and top with a few slices of avocado before serving.

33) Vegetable dish with sesame

Preparation time:

Cooking time:

Portions:

Ingredients:
- ✓ Sesame seeds (1 teaspoon)
- ✓ Lemon juice (.5)
- ✓ Tamari sauce (2 tablespoons)
- ✓ Chopped garlic clove (1)
- ✓ Diced red pepper (.5 c.)

Directions:
- ❖ Heat half a tablespoon of sesame oil and one tablespoon of olive oil in a frying pan. Add the tofu and let it cook for a while.
- ❖ After ten minutes, remove the tofu and add a little more of the two oils.

Ingredients:
- ✓ Finely chopped broccoli florets (2 c.)
- ✓ Cubed tofu (8 oz)
- ✓ Olive oil (2 tablespoons)
- ✓ Sesame oil, toasted (1.5 tbsp)

- ❖ Stir in the garlic, red pepper and broccoli until they soften a little. Add the tofu and also stir in the lemon juice and soy sauce.
- ❖ Top this dish with a few sesame seeds before serving.

34) Sweet spinach salad

Preparation time:

Cooking time:

Portions:

Ingredients:
- ✓ Crushed black pepper (1 teaspoon)
- ✓ Salt (1 teaspoon)
- ✓ Nutmeg (1 teaspoon)
- ✓ Cinnamon (1 teaspoon)
- ✓ Chopped spinach (4 c.)
- ✓ Chopped parsley (2 tablespoons)

Directions:
- ❖ To start this recipe, take out a large bowl and combine all the ingredients together.

Ingredients:
- ✓ Chopped walnuts (.25 c.)
- ✓ Sultanas (.25 c.)
- ✓ Sliced apple (.5 c.)
- ✓ Yoghurt (.5 c.)
- ✓ Lime juice (1 tablespoon)
- ✓ Shredded carrots (.75 c.)
- ❖ Place the bowl in the refrigerator to cool for about ten minutes before serving.

35) Steamed green bowl

Preparation time: **Cooking time:**   **Portions:**

Ingredients:

- ✓ Chopped coriander (2 tbsp)
- ✓ Salt (1 teaspoon)
- ✓ Sliced green onions (2)
- ✓ Ground cashews (1 c.)
- ✓ Coconut milk (2 c.)
- ✓ Green peas (.5 c.)
- ✓ Sliced courgettes (1)

Directions:

- ❖ Heat some coconut oil in a pan and when hot, add the ginger, turmeric, garlic and onion.
- ❖ After five minutes of cooking, add the coconut milk, peas, courgettes and broccoli to this mixture.

Ingredients:

- ✓ Head of broccoli (1)
- ✓ Grated ginger (1 inch)
- ✓ Turmeric (1 teaspoon)
- ✓ Chopped garlic clove (1)
- ✓ Sliced onion (1)
- ✓ Coconut oil (1 tablespoon)

- ❖ Let the ingredients come to the boil before reducing the heat and simmering for a while.
- ❖ After another 15 minutes, stir in the coriander, salt, green onions and cashews before serving.

36) Vegetable and berry salad

Preparation time: **Cooking time:**   **Portions:**

Ingredients:

- ✓ Raspberries (.5 c.)
- ✓ Sliced tangerine (.5)
- ✓ Alfalfa sprouts (1c)
- ✓ Shredded red cabbage (.5 head)
- ✓ Lemon juice 1
- ✓ Olive oil (3 tablespoons)
- ✓ Diced cucumber (1)
- ✓ Avocado (1)
- ✓ Sliced shallot (1)

Directions:

- ❖ Take a large bowl and add all the ingredients.

Ingredients:

- ✓ Sliced cabbage (4 leaves)
- ✓ Chopped parsley (1 tablespoon)
- ✓ Sliced red pepper (.5)
- ✓ Shredded carrot (1)
- ✓ Crushed almonds (1 tablespoon)
- ✓ Pumpkin seeds (2 tablespoons)

- ❖ Stir well to combine before seasoning the fruit and vegetables with a little lemon juice and a little oil.
- ❖ Serve immediately.

37) Bowl of quinoa and carrots

Preparation time: **Cooking time:**   **Portions:**

Ingredients:

- ✓ Sliced green onions (2 tablespoons)
- ✓ Black sesame seeds (2 tablespoons)
- ✓ Salt (.25 tsp.)
- ✓ Chopped parsley (3 tablespoons)
- ✓ Lemon juice (.5)
- ✓ Cooked quinoa (2 c.)

Directions:

- ❖ Whisk together the miso and water in a bowl. Then take a frying pan and heat some oil in it.
- ❖ When the oil is hot, add the fennel bulb and carrots and cook for a few minutes, turning when three minutes have passed.

Ingredients:

- ✓ Sliced fennel bulb (1)
- ✓ Carrots, chopped (1 bunch)
- ✓ Olive oil (1 tablespoon)
- ✓ Miso (1 tablespoon)
- ✓ Water (1 c.)

- ❖ Add the water and miso mixture to the pan and reduce the heat to low. Cook with the lid on for a while. This will take about 20 minutes.
- ❖ While this mixture is cooking, combine the quinoa with the parsley, lemon juice and salt in a bowl.
- ❖ When the carrots are ready, add the mixture on top of the quinoa. Sprinkle the green onions and sesame seeds on top before serving.

38) Grab and Go Wraps

Preparation time:

Cooking time:

Portions:

Ingredients:
- ✓ Carrot cut into julienne strips (1)
- ✓ Red pepper (.5)
- ✓ Chard greens (4)
- ✓ Salt (.25 tsp.)
- ✓ Diced jalapeno pepper (.5)

Directions:
- ❖ Get out your blender or food processor and combine together the salt, jalapeno, shallot, cilantro, lime, avocado and peas. Process to combine, but leave some texture to still be there.

Ingredients:
- ✓ Shallots, diced (1)
- ✓ Chopped coriander leaves (.25 c.)
- ✓ Lime juice (1)
- ✓ Avocado (1)
- ✓ Steamed green peas (1 c.)
- ❖ Spread the collards on the counter and then sprinkle the pea and avocado mixture over them.
- ❖ Add the carrot and pepper strips before rolling up the collars and secure with a toothpick.
- ❖ Repeat with all the ingredients before serving.

39) Walnut tacos

Preparation time:

Cooking time:

Portions:

Ingredients:
- ✓ Chopped coriander (1 tablespoon)
- ✓ Nutritional yeast (2 tablespoons)
- ✓ Romaine lettuce leaves (6)
- ✓ Cooked red quinoa (.25 c.)
- ✓ Salt (.25 tsp.)
- ✓ Tamari (1 tablespoon)
- ✓ Coconut amino acids (1 teaspoon)
- ✓ Smoked paprika (.25 tsp.)

Directions:
- ❖ To start this recipe, add the almonds and walnuts to the food processor and puree them.
- ❖ Add the tomatoes and give a couple of pulses until you have a nice crumbly mixture.
- ❖ From here, add the salt, tamari, coconut aminos, paprika, onion, garlic, chilli, cilantro, cumin and olive oil.

Ingredients:
- ✓ Onion powder (.25 tsp.)
- ✓ Garlic powder (.25 tsp.)
- ✓ Chilli powder (.25 tsp.)
- ✓ Ground coriander (1 teaspoon)
- ✓ Ground cumin (1 teaspoon)
- ✓ Olive oil (2 tablespoons)
- ✓ Chopped dried tomatoes (.25 c.)
- ✓ Chopped raw almonds (.25 c.)
- ✓ Walnuts (.5 c.)
- ❖ It pulses a few more times to be fully combined.
- ❖ Add the tomato and walnut mixture to a bowl and combine with the quinoa.
- ❖ Divide this mixture between the romaine lettuce leaves and top with the coriander and nutritional yeast before serving.

40) Tex-Mex bowl

Preparation time: **Cooking time:**   **Portions:**

Ingredients:
- ✓ Nutritional yeast (2 tablespoons)
- ✓ Cilantro (2 tablespoons)
- ✓ Sliced avocado (1)
- ✓ Salt (.25 tsp.)
- ✓ Olive oil (.25 c.)
- ✓ Apple cider vinegar (.25 c.)
- ✓ Lime juice and zest (1)
- ✓ Lemon juice and zest (1)
- ✓ Squeezed oranges (2)
- ✓ Chopped garlic cloves (2)
- ✓ Sliced red onion (1)
- ✓ Sliced peppers
- ✓ For the brown rice
- ✓ Hind beans (.5 c.)

Directions:
- ❖ Take out a large bowl and combine the salt, olive oil, vinegar, lime zest and juice, lemon zest and juice, garlic, red onion and pepper.
- ❖ Cover and leave for about five hours to marinate a little. While the peppers marinate a bit in the fridge, it's time to work on the sauce.
- ❖ To make the sauce, add all the ingredients to a small bowl and mix well to combine. Cover the bowl and place it in the fridge.

Ingredients:
- ✓ Garlic powder (.5 tsp.)
- ✓ Cayenne pepper (.5 tsp.)
- ✓ Paprika (1 teaspoon)
- ✓ Salt (1 teaspoon)
- ✓ Garlic powder (1.5 teaspoons)
- ✓ Chilli powder (2 teaspoons)
- ✓ Cooked brown rice (1 c.)
- ✓ Salsa
- ✓ Juice of one lime
- ✓ Salt (.25 tsp.)
- ✓ Diced Cilantro (.25 c.)
- ✓ Diced red onion (.5)
- ✓ Diced tomatoes (2)

- ❖ In a medium bowl, add all the ingredients for the brown rice. Mix well and set aside.
- ❖ Heat your frying pan and add the peppers with some of the marinade. Cook for a while until the onion and the peppers are soft.
- ❖ Add the rice to some serving bowls and top with the pepper and onion mixture, salsa and avocado. Add the nutritional yeast and cilantro before serving.

41) Avocado and salmon soup

Preparation time: **Cooking time:**   **Portions:**

Ingredients:
- ✓ Cilantro (2 tablespoons)
- ✓ Crushed pepper (1 teaspoon)
- ✓ Olive oil (1 tablespoon)
- ✓ Salmon flakes (1 can)
- ✓ Salt (.25 tsp.)
- ✓ Cumin (.25 tsp.)
- ✓ Vegetable stock (1.5 c.)

Directions:
- ❖ Take out a blender and combine the salt, cumin, vegetable stock, coconut cream, two tablespoons of lemon juice, green onion, shallot and avocado.
- ❖ Blend until smooth and then chill in the fridge for an hour.

Ingredients:
- ✓ Whole coconut cream (2 tablespoons)
- ✓ Lemon juice (4 tablespoons)
- ✓ Sliced green onion (1 tablespoon)
- ✓ Chopped shallots (1)
- ✓ Pitted avocado (3)

- ❖ Meanwhile, take a bowl and combine one tablespoon of coriander, two tablespoons of lemon juice, pepper, olive oil and the salmon.
- ❖ Add the cooled avocado soup to the bowls and top each with the salmon and the rest of the coriander. Serve immediately.

42) Asian pumpkin salad

Preparation time: **Cooking time:**   **Portions:**

Ingredients:

- ✓ Diced avocado (.5)
- ✓ Pomegranate seeds (.25 c.)
- ✓ Lemon juice (1 tablespoon)
- ✓ Sliced cabbage (4 c.)
- ✓ Olive oil (1.5 tablespoons)
- ✓ Diced pumpkin (2 c.)
- ✓ Salt (.5 tsp.)

Ingredients:

- ✓ Red pepper flakes (.25 tsp.)
- ✓ Ground mustard (.25 tsp.)
- ✓ Ground garlic (.25 tsp.)
- ✓ Ground cloves (.25 tsp.)
- ✓ Black sesame seeds (1 tablespoon)
- ✓ White sesame seeds (1 tablespoon)

Directions:

- ❖ Turn on the oven and give it time to heat up to 400 degrees. Prepare a baking tray with baking paper.
- ❖ In a large dish, combine the black and white sesame seeds with the salt, chilli flakes, mustard, garlic and cloves.
- ❖ Drizzle the pumpkin with a little olive oil and then roll each cube in the sesame seed mixture, pressing a little to coat it.

- ❖ Add the pumpkin to the baking tray and place it in the oven. It will take about half an hour to cook.
- ❖ While the pumpkin is cooking, add the cabbage to a large bowl and pour in the salt, lemon juice and the rest of the olive oil. Massage the mixture into the cabbage and then set aside.
- ❖ When the pumpkin is ready, add it on top of the cabbage and garnish with the avocado and pomegranate seeds before serving.

43) Sweet potato rolls

Preparation time: **Cooking time:**   **Portions:**

Ingredients:

- ✓ Avocado (1)
- ✓ Alfalfa sprouts (1c)
- ✓ Sliced red onion (.5)
- ✓ Spinach (1 c.)
- ✓ Cooked quinoa (.5 c.)
- ✓ Chard greens (4)
- ✓ Sweet potato hummus
- ✓ Crushed black pepper (.25 tsp.)

Ingredients:

- ✓ Salt (.25 tsp.)
- ✓ Cinnamon powder (.25 tsp.)
- ✓ Chilli powder (.25 tsp.)
- ✓ Garlic clove (1)
- ✓ Lemon juice (.5)
- ✓ Olive oil (.25 c.)
- ✓ Tahini (.33 c.)
- ✓ Diced sweet potato (1)
- ❖ Work until the mixture is smooth.
- ❖ Spread each of the green collars and then spread sweet potato hummus on each.
- ❖ Add the avocado, sprouts, onion, spinach and quinoa. Roll everything up and secure with toothpicks. Repeat until the vegetables and filling are finished.

Directions:

- ❖ Take the sweet potatoes and add them to a pan. Cover with water and bring to the boil. When it comes to the boil, reduce the flame and let it cook for a while to make the potatoes tender.
- ❖ When they are ready, drain the water and add them to the food processor together with pepper, salt, cinnamon, chilli powder, garlic, lemon juice, olive oil and tahini.

44) Spicy cabbage bowl

Preparation time: **Cooking time:**   **Portions:**

Ingredients:

- ✓ Sesame seeds (1 tablespoon)
- ✓ Green onion (.25 c.)
- ✓ Cabbage (2 c.)
- ✓ Coconut amino acids (1 teaspoon)
- ✓ Tamari (2 tablespoons)
- ✓ Chopped kimchi cabbage (1 c.)

Ingredients:

- ✓ Cooked brown rice (1 c.)
- ✓ Chopped garlic (1 teaspoon)
- ✓ Grated ginger (.5 tsp.)
- ✓ Sesame oil (2 tablespoons)

- ❖ After five minutes of cooking these ingredients, add the green onions and cabbage and toss to combine.
- ❖ Cook for a little longer. Then you can garnish the dish with sesame seeds before serving.

Directions:

- ❖ Take out a frying pan and heat the sesame oil in it. When the oil is hot, add the coconut amino acid, tamari, kimchi, brown rice, garlic and ginger together.

45) Citrus fruit and fennel salad

Preparation time: Cooking time: Portions:

Ingredients:

- ✓ Diced avocado (.5)
- ✓ Pomegranate seeds (2 tablespoons)
- ✓ Pepper (.5 tsp.)
- ✓ Salt (.25 tsp.)
- ✓ Olive oil (.25 c.)
- ✓ Orange juice (2 tablespoons)
- ✓ Lemon juice (2 tablespoons)

Ingredients:

- ✓ Chopped mint (1 tablespoon)
- ✓ Chopped parsley (.5 c.)
- ✓ Sliced fennel bulbs (2)
- ✓ Red segmented grapefruit (.5)
- ✓ Segmented orange (1)

Directions:

- ❖ To start this recipe, take out a large bowl and combine together the parsley, mint, fennel slices, grapefruit segments and orange segments. Stir to combine.
- ❖ In another bowl, whisk together the pepper, salt, olive oil, orange juice and lemon juice.

- ❖ Once combined, pour over the fennel and citrus mixture in the large bowl, stirring to coat.
- ❖ Move to a plate and garnish with the avocado and pomegranate seeds. Serve immediately.

46) Vegan burger

Preparation time: Cooking time: Servings: 4 hamburger patties

Ingredients:

- ✓ 1/4 to 1/2 cup of spring water
- ✓ 1/2 teaspoon of cayenne powder
- ✓ 1/2 teaspoon of ginger powder
- ✓ Grape oil
- ✓ 1 teaspoon of dill
- ✓ 2 teaspoons of sea salt
- ✓ 2 teaspoons of onion powder

Ingredients:

- ✓ 2 teaspoons of oregano
- ✓ 2 teaspoons of basil
- ✓ ¼ cup cherry tomatoes, diced
- ✓ 1/2 cup of cabbage, diced
- ✓ 1/2 cup green peppers, diced
- ✓ 1/2 cup onions, diced
- ✓ 1 cup of chickpea flour
- ❖ Divide the dough into 4 meatballs. Cook the patties in grapeseed oil in a frying pan over a medium heat for about 2 to 3 minutes per side. Keep turning until the burger is brown on all sides.
- ❖ Serve the burger on a bun and enjoy.

Directions:

- ❖ Mix the vegetables and seasonings in a large bowl, then add the flour. Gently add the spring water and stir the mixture until combined. If the mixture is too soft, add more flour.

47) Alkaline spicy cabbage

Preparation time: Cooking time: Portions: 1 portion

Ingredients:

- ✓ Grape oil
- ✓ 1/4 teaspoon sea salt
- ✓ 1 teaspoon crushed red pepper

Ingredients:

- ✓ 1/4 cup red pepper, diced
- ✓ 1/4 cup onion, diced
- ✓ 1 bunch of cabbage
- ❖ Fry the peppers and onions in oil for about 2-3 minutes and then season with a little sea salt.
- ❖ Lower the heat and add the cabbage, cover the wok with a lid and simmer for about 5 minutes.
- ❖ Open the lid and add the crushed pepper, stir well and cover again. Cook until tender, or for another 3 minutes or so.

Directions:

- ❖ First wash the cabbage well and then fold each cabbage leaf in half. Cut off and discard the stalks. Cut the prepared cabbage into bite-sized portions and use the salad spinner to remove the water.
- ❖ In a wok, add 2 tablespoons of grapeseed oil and heat the oil over high heat.

48) Electric salad

Preparation time: **Cooking time:** **Portions: 4**

Ingredients:

- ✓ 3 jalapenos
- ✓ 2 red onions
- ✓ 1 orange pepper
- ✓ 1 yellow pepper
- ✓ 1 cup cherry tomatoes, chopped

Directions:

- ❖ First wash and rinse the ingredients well. Dry the ingredients and then cut them into bite-size pieces, or as required.

Ingredients:

- ✓ 1 bunch of cabbage
- ✓ 1 handful of romaine lettuce
- ✓ Extra virgin olive oil
- ✓ Juice of 1 lime

- ❖ Put the ingredients in a bowl and drizzle with olive oil and lime juice according to your taste.

49) Kale salad

Preparation time: **Cooking time:** **Portions: 2**

Ingredients:

- ✓ 1/4 teaspoon of cayenne
- ✓ 1/2 teaspoon of sea salt
- ✓ 1/2 cup of cooked chickpeas
- ✓ 1/2 cup red onions
- ✓ 1/2 cup of sliced red, orange, yellow and green peppers
- ✓ 4 cups chopped cabbage

Directions:

- ❖ In a bowl, mix all the ingredients for the coleslaw and stir.

Ingredients:

- ✓ 1/2 cup of alkaline garlic sauce (recipe included).
- ✓ Alkaline garlic sauce
- ✓ 1/4 teaspoon of dill
- ✓ 1/4 teaspoon sea salt
- ✓ 1/2 teaspoon of ginger
- ✓ 1 tablespoon onion powder
- ✓ 1/4 cup shallots, chopped
- ✓ 1 cup of grape oil
- ❖ Prepare the seasoning by mixing the ingredients for the "Alkaline Electric Garlic Sauce".
- ❖ Drizzle with half a cup of sauce and then serve.

50) Walnut, date, orange and cabbage salad

Preparation time: **Cooking time:** **Portions: 2**

Ingredients:

- ✓ /2 red onion, very thinly sliced
- ✓ 2 bunches of cabbage, or 6 full cups of sprouts
- ✓ 6 medjool dates, pitted
- ✓ 1/3 cup whole walnuts
- ✓ For the dressing

Directions:

- ❖ Preheat the oven to 375 degrees F and then place the walnuts on a baking sheet. Roast the walnuts for about 7-8 minutes, or until the skin begins to darken and crack.
- ❖ Once this is done, transfer the nuts while still hot and steam them for 15 minutes wrapped in a kitchen towel.
- ❖ Once cooled, squeeze and turn firmly to remove the skin, still wrapped in the towel.
- ❖ In a food processor, place the pitted dates together with the walnuts and puree until fully mixed and finely chopped. Set aside to cover the salad.

Ingredients:

- ✓ 5 tablespoons of olive oil
- ✓ Pinch of coarse salt
- ✓ 1 medjool date
- ✓ 4 tablespoons of freshly squeezed orange juice
- ✓ 2 tablespoons of lime juice
- ❖ Then wash, dry and cut the cabbage and place it in a large bowl. Thinly slice the onion and add it to the bowl.
- ❖ Now prepare the dressing by combining the ingredients for the "dressing" in the blender, apart from the olive oil.
- ❖ Blend the mixture to break up the dates and then pour in the oil in a steady stream to emulsify the seasoning.
- ❖ Finally, toss the cabbage and onion mixture with the orange and walnut dressing.
- ❖ Move to a serving bowl and sprinkle with the walnut and date mixture. Enjoy your meal!

51) Tomatoes with basil-snack

Preparation time: **Cooking time:**   **Portions: 1 portion**

Ingredients:
- ¼ teaspoon of sea salt
- 2 tablespoons of lemon juice
- 2 tablespoons of olive oil

Directions:
- Start by slicing the cherry tomatoes and placing them in a medium-sized bowl.
- Then finely chop your basil and add it to the bowl of tomatoes.

Ingredients:
- ¼ cup basil, fresh
- 1 cup chopped tomatoes, cherry or Roma

- Sprinkle the tomatoes and basil with a little olive oil and lemon juice.
- Add a little sea salt to taste.
- Serve.

52) Pasta with spelt, courgettes and aubergines

Preparation time: **Cooking time:**   **Portions: 4**

Ingredients:
- 2 teaspoons of dried basil leaves
- 1 teaspoon of oregano
- 2/3 cup vegetable stock
- 2/3 cup of diced, dried cherry tomatoes
- 1 large courgette, diced
- 3 medium-sized, ripe, diced cherry tomatoes

Directions:
- Over a medium heat, heat a little oil in a frying pan and then fry the aubergine, ginger and onion for about 8-10 minutes, stirring constantly.
- Then add the oregano, tomatoes and courgettes and cook for 6-8 minutes, stirring occasionally.

Ingredients:
- 2-3 ginger, crushed
- 1-2 white onions, finely chopped
- 3 tablespoons of cold-pressed extra virgin olive oil
- 1 large diced aubergine
- 300g of spelt pasta
- Sea salt to taste
- Now heat the water and cook the pasta until it is firm to the bite, and then add the vegetable stock to the pan.
- Season with fresh pepper, salt and dried basil. Leave the mixture to simmer for a few minutes, covered.
- Once cooked, you can serve the sauce over pasta and garnish with fresh basil leaves.

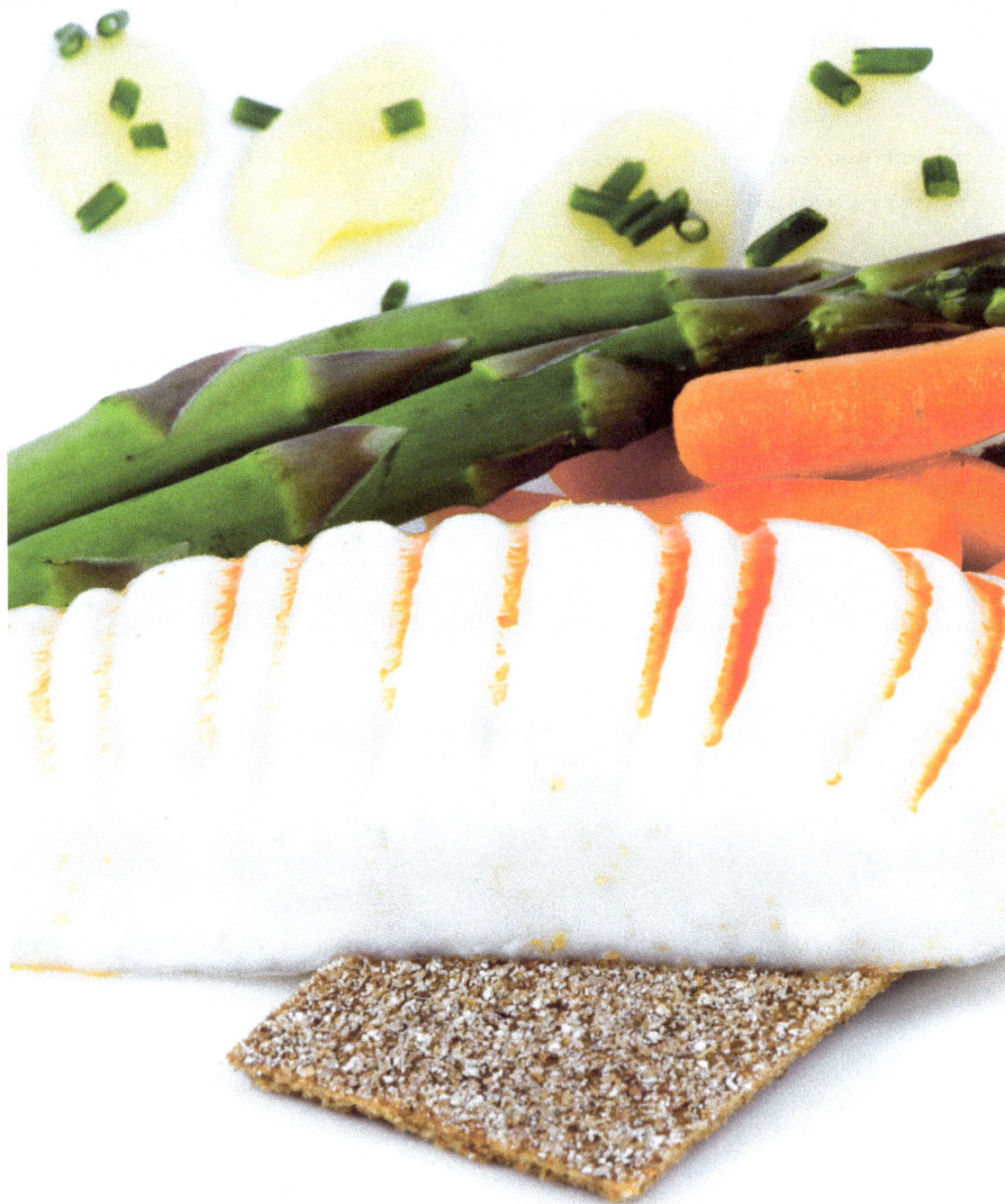

53) Stew without beef

Preparation time: **Cooking time:**   **Portions: 4**

Ingredients:
- ✓ Dried oregano, 1 teaspoon
- ✓ Celery, diced, 2 stalks
- ✓ Large diced potato
- ✓ Sliced carrot, 3 c.
- ✓ Water, 2 c.
- ✓ Vegetable stock, 3 c.

Ingredients:
- ✓ Pepper, one teaspoon
- ✓ Sea salt, one teaspoon
- ✓ Garlic puree, 2 bulbs
- ✓ Diced onion, 1 c.
- ✓ Avocado oil, 1 tablespoon
- ✓ Laurel
- ❖ Taste and adjust the seasonings as necessary. If it is too thick, you can add more water or stock.
- ❖ Divide between four bowls and enjoy.

Directions:
- ❖ Heat the avocado oil in an upper pan. Add the pepper, salt, garlic cloves and onion bulbs. Cook everything for two to three minutes, or until the onion is soft.
- ❖ Add the bay leaf, oregano, celery, potato, carrot, water and stock. Let it simmer, then turn down the heat and cook for 30-45 minutes, or until the carrots and potatoes are soft.

54) Emmenthal soup

Preparation time: **Cooking time:**   **Portions: 2**

Ingredients:
- ✓ Cayenne
- ✓ Nutmeg
- ✓ Pumpkin seeds, 1 tablespoon
- ✓ Chopped chives, 2 tablespoons

Ingredients:
- ✓ Diced Emmenthal cheese, 3 tablespoons
- ✓ Vegetable stock, 2 c.
- ✓ Diced potato, 1
- ✓ Chopped cauliflower, 2 c.
- ❖ Add the spices and adjust to taste.
- ❖ Pour into bowls, add the chives and cheese and mix well.
- ❖ Garnish with pumpkin seeds. Enjoy your meal.

Directions:
- ❖ Put the potato and cauliflower in a saucepan with the vegetable stock until tender.
- ❖ Place in a blender and blend.

55) Spaghetti with broccoli

Preparation time: **Cooking time:**   **Portions: 2**

Ingredients:
- ✓ Pepe
- ✓ Halls
- ✓ Vegetable stock, 1 teaspoon
- ✓ Oregano plant, 1 teaspoon
- ✓ Lemon juice, 1 tablespoon
- ✓ Sliced carrots, 3
- ✓ Diced tomatoes, 3

Ingredients:
- ✓ Broccoli cut into florets, 1 head
- ✓ Sliced red pepper - bell, one
- ✓ Sliced onion bulb, one
- ✓ Diced garlic bulbs, two cloves
- ✓ EVOO, 4 tablespoons
- ✓ Buckwheat paste, 1 lb.

Directions:
- ❖ Put a pot of water halfway up and add salt. Let it boil and add the pasta. Prepare according to the instructions on the tin. Empty.
- ❖ Place the broccoli in another bowl and cover with h2O. Prepare for five minutes.
- ❖ Place a frying pan over normal heat and put two tablespoons of olive oil in the pan and heat. Put the bulbs, garlic and onion in and cook until soft and fragrant. Remove from the pan and set aside.

- ❖ carrots. Cook for five minutes, then put on the sweet pepper and prepare for another five minutes, now put on the tomatoes and prepare for two minutes.
- ❖ Drain the broccoli completely and add it to the pan with the rest of the vegetables. Put the onions and garlic back into the pan.
- ❖ Add the vegetable stock, oregano and lemon juice. Add a little pepper and salt, taste and adjust seasonings if necessary. Stir well to combine.
- ❖ Place the cooked pasta on a serving plate. Pour in the vegetable mixture and stir.

56) Indian Lentil Curry

Preparation time: **Cooking time:**   **Portions: 4 - 6**

Ingredients:
- ✓ Lime juice
- ✓ Chopped coriander
- ✓ Halls
- ✓ EVOO, 1 tablespoon
- ✓ Diced tomatoes, 2
- ✓ Sliced onion, 1

Directions:
- ❖ Put the lentils in a bowl, cover with water and leave to stand for six hours.
- ❖ After six hours, drain the lentils completely.
- ❖ Place a bowl over normal heat. Put the lentils in and cover with fresh water. Leave to boil. Add the turmeric. Lower the heat and simmer until the lentils are cooked.
- ❖ Remove from the pan and place in a bowl. Set aside.

Ingredients:
- ✓ Chopped garlic, 1 clove
- ✓ Grated ginger, 1 inch
- ✓ Turmeric, .5 tsp
- ✓ Cumin seeds, .5 tsp
- ✓ Chopped green peppers, 2
- ✓ Fine red lentils, 1 c.
- ❖ In another pan over medium heat, heat the olive oil. Add the turmeric, cumin, ginger and onions. Cook until the onions are soft and the ginger is fragrant.
- ❖ Add the chillies and tomatoes and cook. Add salt and cook for five minutes.
- ❖ Pour the lentil into this mixture and bring back to a simmer. As soon as it starts to cook, remove it from the hot temperature. Squeeze a little lemon
- ❖ Sprinkle with coriander and serve with rice.

57) Vegetables with wild rice

Preparation time: **Cooking time:**   **Portions: 4**

Ingredients:
- ✓ Halls
- ✓ Basil
- ✓ Cilantro
- ✓ Juice of one lime
- ✓ Chopped red pepper, 1
- ✓ Vegetable stock, .5 c.

Directions:
- ❖ Put all the chopped vegetables in a pan and add the vegetable stock.
- ❖ Steam-fry the vegetables until they are cooked but still crispy.

Ingredients:
- ✓ Bean sprouts, 1 c.
- ✓ Chopped carrots, 2 c.
- ✓ Beans - green - diced, 1 c.
- ✓ Broccoli, cut, 1 c.
- ✓ Pak Choi, 1 c.
- ✓ Wild rice, 1 c.
- ❖ Using a mortar and pestle, grind the chilli, basil and coriander to a paste. Add the lime juice and mix well.
- ❖ Place the rice on a serving plate. Add the vegetables on top and drizzle with the dressing.

58) Spicy lentil soup

Preparation time: **Cooking time:**   **Portions: 4**

Ingredients:
- ✓ Halls
- ✓ Turmeric, .25 tsp
- ✓ Chopped garlic, 3 cloves
- ✓ Grated ginger, 1.5 inch piece
- ✓ Chopped tomato, 1

Directions:
- ❖ Put the lentils in a colander and place them under running water. Rinse until the soil and stones are removed.
- ❖ Pour the rinsed lentils into a pot. Add enough water to cover the lentils. Put the pot over medium heat and let it boil.

Ingredients:
- ✓ Chopped Serrano chilli pepper, 1
- ✓ Rinsed red lentils, 2 c.
- ✓ Topping:
- ✓ Coconut yoghurt, .25 c.

- ❖ Lower the heat and simmer for ten minutes.
- ❖ Put in the contents of the leftovers and then mix well to combine.
- ❖ Cook again until the lentils are soft.
- ❖ Garnish with a spoonful of coconut yoghurt.

59) Leek soup with mushrooms

Preparation time: Cooking time: Portions: 4

Ingredients:

- ✓ Sherry vinegar, 1.5 tablespoons
- ✓ Almond milk, .5 c.
- ✓ Coconut cream, .66 c.
- ✓ Vegetable stock, 3 c.
- ✓ Chopped dill, 1 tablespoon
- ✓ Pepe
- ✓ Halls

Ingredients:

- ✓ Almond flour, 5 tablespoons
- ✓ Cleaned and sliced mushrooms, 7 c.
- ✓ Chopped garlic, 3 cloves
- ✓ Chopped leeks, 2.75 c.
- ✓ Vegetable oil, 3 tablespoons

Directions:

- ❖ Set a Dutch oven to medium and heat the oil. Add the leeks and bulb garlic and cook until soft.
- ❖ Add the mushrooms, stir and cook for another 10 minutes.

- ❖ Add the salt, dill, pepper and flour. Mix well, until combined.
- ❖ Put the soup in and let it simmer. Reduce the heat and add the rest of the ingredients. Stir well. Cook for another ten minutes.
- ❖ Serve hot with almond flour bread.

60) Fresh vegetarian pizza

Preparation time: Cooking time: Portions: 4

Ingredients:

-   Crust -
- ✓ Garlic bulb flavoured powder, 0.5 teaspoon
- ✓ Sea salt, 0.5 teaspoon
- ✓ Coconut oil, 3 tablespoons
- ✓ Almond flour, 1.25 c.
- ✓ Tahini-Bee Spread -
- ✓ Pepper, pinch

Ingredients:

- ✓ Sea salt, a pinch
- ✓ Garlic, 2 cloves
- ✓ Lemon juice, one tablespoon
- ✓ Avocado oil, one tablespoon
- ✓ Middle Eastern pasta, one tablespoon
- ✓ Peeled and diced beets, 2

Directions:

- ❖ Start by setting your oven to 375. Place some parchment on a tray.
- ❖ Mix together the salt, garlic powder, coconut oil and almond flour.
- ❖ Place it on the tray and flatten it into a ball shape. Place another piece of parchment on top and roll out the dough into a 7x7 square. Bake for 14 minutes, or until it starts to brown.

- ❖ While the crust is cooking, add the pepper, salt, garlic, lemon juice, avocado oil, tahini and beetroot to a food processor. Blend until creamy.
- ❖ To make your pizza, spread the crust with beetroot sauces and then top with your favourite alkaline friendly vegetables. Cut it into four and enjoy.

61) Spicy lentil burger

Preparation time: Cooking time: Portions: 4

Ingredients:

- ✓ Avocado oil, 1 tablespoon
- ✓ Coconut flour, 1 tablespoon
- ✓ Crushed garlic, 2 cloves
- ✓ Jalapeno cubes
- ✓ Crushed cilantro, .5 c.

Directions:

- ❖ Cook the lentils according to the packet instructions and set aside to cool.
- ❖ Mix together the garlic, jalapeno, cilantro, onion, pepper, salt, almond flour and lentils until well combined.
- ❖ Add half of the lentil mixture to a food processor and process until it reaches a paste-like consistency.
- ❖ Pour this into the bowl with the rest of the lentil mixture and mix everything together.

Ingredients:

- ✓ Diced onion, .5 c.
- ✓ Pepper, .5 tsp
- ✓ Sea salt, 0.5 teaspoons
- ✓ Almond flour, .5 c.
- ✓ Dried lentils, .5 c.
- ❖ The mixture will be very moist. Stir in the coconut flour to help get rid of the moisture and to help hold it together.
- ❖ Divide the mixture into quarters. Squeeze a quarter of the mixture between your hands to flatten it into a hamburger shape. Do this for the remaining three sections.
- ❖ Heat the oil in a large frying pan and place the burgers in it. Cook the burgers for 4 to 6 minutes on both sides, or until golden brown. When flipping them, do so carefully so they don't fall apart. Enjoy your meal.

62) Roasted cauliflower rolls

Preparation time: **Cooking time:**   **Portions: 2**

Ingredients:

- ✓ Cauliflower -
- ✓ Pepper, .25 tsp
- ✓ Sea salt, .25 tsp
- ✓ Garlic powder, .5 tsp
- ✓ Nutritional yeast, .25 c.
- ✓ Almond flour, .25 c.
- ✓ Avocado oil, 1 tablespoon
- ✓ Bitten cauliflower florets, 2 c.
- ✓ Salsa -
- ✓ Sea salt

Directions:

- ❖ Start by setting your kitchen appliance to three hundred and fifty degrees and then put some paper on a kitchen wrap.
- ❖ To prepare the cauliflower, toss it in the avocado oil and make sure it is evenly coated.
- ❖ In a container, combine all the seasonings: pepper, salt, garlic powder, healthy mushrooms, together with the almond flour.
- ❖ Sprinkle the breading over the cauliflower and toss, making sure the cauliflower is well coated. Spread on the baking tray.

Ingredients:

- ✓ Apple cider vinegar, 2 tablespoons
- ✓ Garlic, 2 cloves
- ✓ Habanero pepper
- ✓ Mango cubes, 1 c.
- ✓ Assembly -
- ✓ Canola shoots, 2 leaves
- ✓ Mixed salad, 1 c.

- ❖ Cook for thirty to thirty-five minutes, or until the cauliflower is soft.
- ❖ While the cauliflower is cooking, add the salt, vinegar, garlic, habanero and mango to your blender and blend until well combined. Be sure to use gloves or wash your hands thoroughly when handling the habanero.
- ❖ To assemble, divide the salad mix between the collard leaves, cover with the cauliflower and pour the sauce over it. Wrap the whole thing like a burrito and enjoy.

63) Sliced sweet potato with creamed artichokes and peppers

Preparation time: **Cooking time:**   **Portions: 4**

Ingredients:

- ✓ Pepper, .25 tsp
- ✓ Salt, .5 tsp
- ✓ Avocado oil, 6 tablespoons - divided
- ✓ Red pepper cut into quarters

Directions:

- ❖ Start by setting the oven to 350. Place some parchment on a tray and set aside.
- ❖ Spread the pepper and sweet potato on the sheet tray and cover with two teaspoons of avocado oil, a pinch of pepper and a pinch of salt.

Ingredients:

- ✓ Unpeeled sweet potatoes, 2 cut into 4 slices lengthwise
- ✓ Garlic, 2 cloves
- ✓ Artichoke hearts, 14 oz can

- ❖ Bake for 30 minutes. Turn them over and bake for a further 15 minutes.
- ❖ Add the roasted red pepper to a food processor along with the garlic, artichoke hearts, pepper, salt and remaining avocado oil. Pulse until combined but still somewhat chunky. Adjust seasonings as needed.
- ❖ Cover the sweet potato slices with the cream and enjoy.

64) Cooking scallops, onions and potatoes

Preparation time: **Cooking time:**   **Portions: 4**

Ingredients:
- Cashew-cheese sauce -
- Sea salt, 0.5 teaspoons
- Nutritional yeast, .5 c.
- Almond milk, 1 c.
- Raw cashews, 1 c.
- Scallop Bake -
- Finely chopped tarragon, 1 tablespoon

Directions:
- To make the cheese sauce, add the cashews to a bowl and cover with room temperature water. Let them soak for 15-20 minutes and then drain and rinse them.
- Blend together the cashews with the remaining cheese sauce ingredients until smooth and creamy. Set aside until later.
- Start by heating the oven to 375.
- Combine the onions and potatoes in a bowl with the avocado oil. Add the tarragon, pepper and salt, making sure everything is well coated.

Ingredients:
- Pepper, 1 teaspoon
- Sea salt, one teaspoon
- Oil - Avocado, one tablespoon
- Chopped small onion bulbs, 1.5
- New potatoes, thinly sliced, 8

- Using an 8-inch square baking dish, place the potato and onion mixture in the dish. Do your best to arrange them in nice rows. It doesn't have to be perfect.
- Bake for 45 minutes, or until the potatoes are soft.
- Remove from the oven and cover with the cheese sauce. Divide between four plates and enjoy. You can also slide this on, and bake inside the cooking appliance on about 5 minutes in order to warm the cheese sauce through before serving.

65) Spicy cilantro and coconut soup

Preparation time: **Cooking time:**   **Portions: 2**

Ingredients:
- Cilantro leaves, 2 tablespoons
- Jalapeno
- Lime juice, 1 tablespoon
- Whole coconut milk, 13.5 oz can

Directions:
- Add the avocado oil to a medium frying pan and heat. Add the salt, garlic and onion and cook for three to five minutes, or until the onion bulbs become smooth.

Ingredients:
- Sea salt, .25 tsp
- Crushed garlic, 3 cloves
- Diced onion, .5 c.
- Avocado oil, 2 tablespoons
- Place the onion mixture, coriander, jalapeno, lime juice and coconut milk in a blender and blend until creamy.
- Pour into a bowl and enjoy.

66) Tarragon soup

Preparation time: **Cooking time:**   **Portions: 2**

Ingredients:
- Chopped fresh tarragon, 2 tablespoons
- Celery stalk
- Raw cashews, .5 c.
- Lemon juice, 1 tablespoon
- Whole coconut milk, 13.5 oz can

Directions:
- Add the oil to a medium frying pan and heat it up. Put all the seasonings: pepper, salt, garlic bulbs, together with the onion bulbs then prepare about three to five minutes, or until the onions become soft.

Ingredients:
- Pepper, .5 tsp - divided
- Sea salt, .5 tsp - divided
- Crushed garlic, 3 cloves
- Diced onion, .5 c.
- Avocado oil, 1 tablespoon
- Using a high-speed blender, add the onion mixture, tarragon, celery, cashews, lemon juice and coconut milk. Blend until smooth. Taste and adjust seasonings if necessary.
- Divide between two bowls and enjoy. You can also add it back into a pot and reheat it before serving.

67) Asparagus and artichoke soup

Preparation time: **Cooking time:**   **Portions: 4**

Ingredients:

- ✓ Artichoke hearts halved and chopped, 1 tin
- ✓ Almond milk, 2 c.
- ✓ Pepper, .5 tsp
- ✓ Sea salt, .5 - .75 tsp
- ✓ Vegetable stock, 2 c.
- ✓ Diced asparagus, 8 stalks

Directions:

- ❖ Add the garlic, avocado oil and onion to a frying pan and cook for a few minutes, or until the onion bulbs have softened and weakened.
- ❖ Put the cooked vegetables in a pot and add pepper, salt, vegetable stock, asparagus and potatoes. Stir everything together and leave to simmer. Lower the heat and simmer gently for eighteen to twenty minutes, or until the potatoes have become soft.

Ingredients:

- ✓ Cubed potatoes, 1 c.
- ✓ Crushed garlic, 2 cloves
- ✓ Avocado oil, 1 tablespoon
- ✓ Diced onion, .5 c.

- ❖ Add a little more stock if you need it, so that the liquid remains about a centimetre above the vegetables.
- ❖ Place the pan away from the heat and allow it to cool.
- ❖ Using a blender, blend the cooled soup with the artichokes and almond milk until everything is well combined and smooth. Adjust the seasonings as necessary. You can add more broth or milk to thicken everything if necessary.
- ❖ Pour back into the pan and leave to heat over a low heat until ready to serve.

68) Mint and berry soup

Preparation time: **Cooking time:**   **Portions: 1**

Ingredients:

- ✓ Sweetener -
- ✓ Water, .25 c - more if necessary
- ✓ Unrefined whole cane sugar, .25 c.
  Soup -
- ✓ Water, .5 c.

Directions:

- ❖ Add the water and sugar to a small saucepan and cook, stirring constantly, until the sugar has dissolved. Leave to cool.
- ❖ Add the mint leaves, lemon juice, water, berries and cooled sugar mixture to a blender. Blend until smooth.

Ingredients:

- ✓ Mixed berries, 1 c.
- ✓ Mint leaves, 8
- ✓ Lemon juice, 1 teaspoon

- ❖ Pour into a bowl and then refrigerate until the broth is completely cooled. This will take about 20 minutes.
- ❖ Have fun.

69) Mushroom soup

Preparation time: **Cooking time:**   **Portions: 2**

Ingredients:

- ✓ Whole coconut milk, 13.5 oz can
- ✓ Vegetable stock, 1 tbsp.
- ✓ Pepper, .5 tsp
- ✓ Sea salt, .75 tsp
- ✓ Crush the garlic clove
- ✓ Diced onion, 1 cup

Directions:

- ❖ Heat the fat in a very large pan, then put all the seasonings: pepper, salt, garlic, onion bulb and mushrooms. Boil and cook for a few minutes, or until the onions are soft.
- ❖ Mix the coconut amino acid, thyme, coconut milk and vegetable stock.

Ingredients:

- ✓ Cut cremini mushrooms, 1 cup
- ✓ Chinese black mushrooms cut into pieces, one cup
- ✓ Avocado oil, 1 tablespoon
- ✓ Coconut amino acids, 1 tablespoon
- ✓ Dried thyme, .5 tsp

- ❖ Lower the heat and let the broth simmer for about fifteen minutes. Stir the broth from time to time.
- ❖ Taste and adjust the seasoning as required. Divide between two bowls and enjoy.

70) Potato and lentil stew

Preparation time: **Cooking time:**   **Portions:** 4

Ingredients:

- ✓ Chopped oregano, 2 sprigs
- ✓ Diced celery stalk
- ✓ Potato, diced and peeled, 1 c.
- ✓ Sliced carrots, 2
- ✓ Dried lentils, 1 c.
- ✓ Spicy seasoning / Pepper, one teaspoon
- ✓ Sea salt, one to 1.5 teaspoons

Directions:

- ❖ Using a large cooking utensil, heat the avocado fat along with the inclusion of seasonings: pepper, salt, garlic bulbs, along with the onion. Cook for three to five minutes, or until the onion is soft.
- ❖ Add the tarragon, oregano, celery, potato, carrots, lentils and 2 ½ cups of vegetable stock. Stir everything together.

Ingredients:

- ✓ Crushed garlic bulbs, two buds
- ✓ Diced onion, .5 c.
- ✓ Avocado oil, 2 tablespoons
- ✓ Whole coconut milk, 13.5 oz can
- ✓ Vegetable stock, 5 c - divided
- ✓ Chopped tarragon, 2 sprigs

- ❖ Allow the saucepan to warm up again and then lower the heat. Leave to cook, stirring frequently. Add more vegetable stock in half-cup portions, if necessary, to make sure the lentils have enough liquid to cook. Let the stew cook for 20-25 minutes, or until the lentils and potatoes are soft.
- ❖ Remove the stew from the heat and stir in the coconut milk. Divide between four bowls and enjoy.

71) Mixed mushroom stew

Preparation time: 15 minutes   **Cooking time:** 15 minutes   **Portions:** 4

Ingredients:

- ✓ 2 tablespoons of olive oil
- ✓ 2 onions, chopped
- ✓ 3 cloves of garlic, minced
- ✓ ½ pound fresh mushrooms, chopped
- ✓ ¼ pound fresh shiitake mushrooms, chopped

Directions:

- ❖ In a large frying pan, heat the oil over medium heat and fry the onion and garlic for 4-5 minutes.
- ❖ Add the mushrooms, salt and black pepper and cook for 4-5 minutes.

Ingredients:

- ✓ ¼ pound fresh Portobello mushrooms, chopped
- ✓ Sea salt and freshly ground black pepper, to taste
- ✓ ¼ cup of homemade vegetable stock
- ✓ ½ cup unsweetened coconut milk
- ✓ 2 tablespoons fresh parsley, chopped
- ❖ Add the broth and coconut milk and bring to a gentle boil.
- ❖ Simmer for 4-5 minutes or until cooked through.
- ❖ Add the parsley and remove from the heat.
- ❖ Serve hot.

72) Mixed spicy vegetable stew

Preparation time: 20 minutes   **Cooking time:** 35 minutes   **Portions:** 8

Ingredients:

- ✓ 2 tablespoons of coconut oil
- ✓ 1 large sweet onion, chopped
- ✓ 1 medium parsnip, peeled and chopped
- ✓ 3 tablespoons of home-made tomato paste
- ✓ 2 large cloves of garlic, minced
- ✓ ½ teaspoon cinnamon powder
- ✓ ½ teaspoon ground ginger
- ✓ 1 teaspoon ground cumin
- ✓ ¼ teaspoon cayenne pepper

Directions:

- ❖ In a large soup pot, melt the coconut oil over medium-high heat and sauté the onion for about 5 minutes.
- ❖ Add the parsnips and fry for about 3 minutes.
- ❖ Add the tomato paste, garlic and spices and fry for 2 minutes.

Ingredients:

- ✓ 2 medium-sized carrots, peeled and chopped
- ✓ 2 medium purple potatoes, peeled and cut into pieces
- ✓ 2 medium sweet potatoes, peeled and cut into pieces
- ✓ 4 cups of homemade vegetable stock
- ✓ 2 tablespoons fresh lemon juice
- ✓ 2 cups fresh cabbage, hard ribs removed and chopped
- ✓ ¼ cup fresh parsley leaves, chopped

- ❖ Stir in the carrots, potatoes, sweet potatoes and stock and bring to the boil.
- ❖ Reduce the heat to medium-low and simmer, covered, for about 20 minutes.
- ❖ Add the lemon juice and the cabbage and simmer for 5 minutes.
- ❖ Serve with a garnish of parsley.

73) Mixed vegetable stew with herbs

Preparation time: 15 minutes   **Cooking time**: 2¼ hours   **Portions**: 8

Ingredients:

- ✓ 2 tablespoons of coconut oil
- ✓ 1 medium yellow onion, chopped
- ✓ 2 cups celery, chopped
- ✓ ½ teaspoon chopped garlic
- ✓ 3 cups fresh cabbage, hard ribs removed and chopped
- ✓ ½ cup fresh mushrooms, sliced
- ✓ 2½ cups tomatoes, finely chopped
- ✓ 1 teaspoon dried rosemary, crushed

Directions:

- ❖ In a large frying pan, melt the coconut oil over medium heat and fry the onion, celery and garlic for about 5 minutes.
- ❖ Add the rest of all the ingredients and stir to combine.
- ❖ Increase the heat to high and bring to the boil.
- ❖ Cook for about 10 minutes.

Ingredients:

- ✓ 1 teaspoon dried sage, crushed
- ✓ 1 teaspoon dried oregano, crushed
- ✓ Sea salt and freshly ground black pepper, to taste
- ✓ 2 cups of homemade vegetable stock
- ✓ 3-4 cups of alkaline water
- ✓ ¼ cup fresh parsley, chopped

- ❖ Reduce the heat to medium and cook, covered, for about 15 minutes.
- ❖ Uncover the pan and cook for about 15 minutes, stirring occasionally.
- ❖ Now reduce the heat to low and simmer, covered, for about 1½ hours.
- ❖ Serve hot with a garnish of parsley.

74) Tofu and pepper stew

Preparation time: 15 minutes   **Cooking time**: 15 minutes   **Portions**: 6

Ingredients:

- ✓ 2 tablespoons of garlic
- ✓ 1 jalapeño pepper, seeded and chopped
- ✓ 1 (16-ounce) jar of roasted, rinsed, drained and chopped red peppers
- ✓ 2 cups of homemade vegetable stock
- ✓ 2 cups of alkaline water

Directions:

- ❖ In a food processor, add the garlic, jalapeño pepper and roasted red peppers and pulse until smooth.
- ❖ In a large pan, add the pepper puree, stock and water over medium-high heat and bring to the boil.
- ❖ Add the peppers and tofu and stir to combine.

Ingredients:

- ✓ 1 medium green pepper, seeded and thinly sliced
- ✓ 1 medium red pepper, seeded and thinly sliced
- ✓ 1 (16-ounce) packet of extra-firm tofu, drained and diced
- ✓ 10 ounces of frozen, thawed sprouts
- ✓ Sea salt and freshly ground black pepper, to taste
- ❖ Reduce the heat to medium and cook for about 5 minutes.
- ❖ Stir in the cabbage and cook for about 5 minutes.
- ❖ Add salt and black pepper and remove from the heat.
- ❖ Serve hot.

75) Roasted pumpkin curry

Preparation time: 15 minutes   **Cooking time**: 35 minutes   **Portions**: 4

Ingredients:

For the roasted pumpkin:
- ✓ 1 medium-sized sugar pumpkin, peeled and cut into cubes
- ✓ Sea salt, to taste
- ✓ 1 teaspoon of olive oil

For Curry:
- ✓ 1 teaspoon of olive oil
- ✓ 1 onion, chopped
- ✓ 1 tablespoon fresh ginger root, peeled and chopped

Directions:

- ❖ Preheat the oven to 400 degrees F. Line a large baking tray with baking paper.
- ❖ In a large bowl, add all the ingredients for the roasted pumpkin and stir to coat well.
- ❖ Arrange the pumpkins on the prepared baking tray in a single layer.
- ❖ Roast for about 20-25 minutes, turning once halfway through.

Ingredients:

- ✓ 1 tablespoon chopped garlic
- ✓ 1 cup unsweetened coconut milk
- ✓ 2 cups of vegetable stock
- ✓ 1 teaspoon ground cumin
- ✓ ½ teaspoon ground turmeric
- ✓ Sea salt and freshly ground black pepper, to taste
- ✓ 1 tablespoon fresh lime juice
- ✓ 2 tablespoons fresh parsley, chopped
- ❖ Meanwhile, for the curry: in a large frying pan, heat the oil over medium-high heat and fry the onion for about 4-5 minutes.
- ❖ Add the ginger and garlic and fry for about 1 minute.
- ❖ Add the coconut milk, broth, spices, salt and black pepper and bring to the boil.
- ❖ Reduce the heat to low and simmer for about 10 minutes.
- ❖ Add the roasted pumpkin and simmer for a further 10 minutes.
- ❖ Serve hot with a garnish of parsley.

76) Lentils, vegetables and apples in curry sauce

Preparation time: 20 minutes **Cooking time**: 1 ½ hours **Portions**: 6

Ingredients:

- ✓ 8 cups of alkaline water
- ✓ ½ teaspoon ground turmeric
- ✓ 1 cup brown lentils
- ✓ 1 cup red lentils
- ✓ 1 tablespoon olive oil
- ✓ 1 large white onion, chopped
- ✓ 3 cloves of garlic, minced
- ✓ 2 tomatoes, seeded and chopped

Directions:

- ❖ In a large pan, add the water, turmeric and lentils over high heat and bring to the boil.
- ❖ Reduce the heat to medium-low and simmer, covered, for about 30 minutes.
- ❖ Drain the lentils, reserving 2½ cups of the cooking liquid.
- ❖ Meanwhile, in another large frying pan, heat the oil over medium heat and fry the onion for about 2-3 minutes.
- ❖ Add the garlic and fry for about 1 minute.
- ❖ Add the tomatoes and cook for about 5 minutes.

Ingredients:

- ✓ ¼ teaspoon of ground cloves
- ✓ 2 teaspoons of ground cumin
- ✓ 2 carrots, peeled and cut into pieces
- ✓ 2 potatoes, peeled and cut into pieces
- ✓ 2 cups of pumpkin, peeled, seeded and cut into 1-inch cubes
- ✓ 1 granny smith apple, cored and chopped
- ✓ 2 cups fresh cabbage, hard ribs removed and chopped
- ✓ Sea salt and freshly ground black pepper, to taste
- ❖ Stir in the spices and cook for about 1 minute.
- ❖ Add the carrots, potatoes, pumpkin, cooked lentils and the reserved cooking liquid and bring to a gentle boil.
- ❖ Reduce the heat to medium-low and simmer, covered, for about 40-45 minutes or until the desired doneness of the vegetables.
- ❖ Add the apple and cabbage and simmer for about 15 minutes.
- ❖ Add salt and black pepper and remove from the heat.
- ❖ Serve hot.

77) Curried red beans

Preparation time: 15 minutes **Cooking time**: 25 minutes **Portions**: 6

Ingredients:

- ✓ 4 tablespoons of olive oil
- ✓ 1 medium onion, finely chopped
- ✓ 2 cloves of garlic, minced
- ✓ 2 tablespoons fresh ginger root, peeled and chopped
- ✓ 1 teaspoon ground coriander
- ✓ 1 teaspoon ground cumin
- ✓ ½ teaspoon ground turmeric

Directions:

- ❖ In a large frying pan, heat the oil over medium heat and fry the onion, garlic and ginger for about 6-8 minutes.
- ❖ Stir in the spices and cook for about 1-2 minutes.

Ingredients:

- ✓ ¼ teaspoon cayenne pepper
- ✓ Sea salt and freshly ground black pepper, to taste
- ✓ 2 large plum tomatoes, finely chopped
- ✓ 3 cups of cooked red beans
- ✓ 2 cups of alkaline water
- ✓ ¼ cup fresh parsley, chopped

- ❖ Add the tomatoes, beans and water and bring to the boil over high heat.
- ❖ Reduce heat to medium and simmer for 10-15 minutes or until desired thickness.
- ❖ Serve hot with a garnish of parsley.

78) Lentil and carrot chili

Preparation time: 15 minutes **Cooking time**: 2 hours 40 minutes **Portions**: 8

Ingredients:

- ✓ 2 teaspoons of olive oil
- ✓ 1 large onion, chopped
- ✓ 3 medium-sized carrots, peeled and chopped
- ✓ 4 celery stalks, chopped
- ✓ 2 cloves of garlic, minced
- ✓ ● 1 jalapeño pepper, seeded and chopped
- ✓ ½ tablespoon dried thyme, crushed
- ✓ 1 tablespoon chipotle chilli powder

Directions:

- ❖ In a large frying pan, heat the oil over medium heat and fry the onion, carrot and celery for about 5 minutes.
- ❖ Add the garlic, jalapeño pepper, thyme and spices and fry for about 1 minute.

Ingredients:

- ✓ ½ tablespoon cayenne pepper
- ✓ 1½ tablespoons ground coriander
- ✓ 1½ tablespoons of ground cumin
- ✓ 1 teaspoon ground turmeric
- ✓ Sea salt and freshly ground black pepper, to taste
- ✓ 1 pound red lentils, rinsed
- ✓ 8 cups of homemade vegetable stock
- ✓ ½ cup shallots, chopped

- ❖ Add the lentils and stock and bring to the boil.
- ❖ Reduce the heat to low and simmer, covered, for about 2-2½ hours.
- ❖ Remove from the heat and serve hot with a shallot garnish.

79) Black beans with chilli

Preparation time: 15 minutes   **Cooking time:** 2 hours and 5 minutes   **Portions: 5**

Ingredients:

- ✓ 2 tablespoons of olive oil
- ✓ 1 onion, chopped
- ✓ 1 large green pepper, seeded and sliced
- ✓ 4 cloves of garlic, minced
- ✓ 2 jalapeño peppers, sliced
- ✓ 1 teaspoon ground cumin
- ✓ 1 teaspoon cayenne pepper

Directions:

- ❖ In a large frying pan, heat the oil over medium-high heat and fry the onion and peppers for 3-4 minutes.
- ❖ Add the garlic, jalapeño peppers and spices and fry for about 1 minute.
- ❖ Add the remaining ingredients and bring to the boil.

Ingredients:

- ✓ 1 tablespoon of red chilli powder
- ✓ 1 teaspoon of paprika
- ✓ 2 cups of tomatoes, finely chopped
- ✓ 4 cups of cooked black beans
- ✓ 2 cups of homemade vegetable stock
- ✓ Sea salt and freshly ground black pepper, to taste
- ✓ ¼ cup fresh parsley, chopped
- ❖ Reduce the heat to medium-low and simmer, covered, for about 1½-2 hours.
- ❖ Season with salt and black pepper and remove from the heat.
- ❖ Serve hot with a garnish of parsley.

80) Cooking mixed vegetables

Preparation time: 15 minutes   **Cooking time:** 20 minutes   **Portions: 4**

Ingredients:

- ✓ 1 small courgette, chopped
- ✓ 1 small summer squash, chopped
- ✓ 1 diced aubergine
- ✓ 1 red pepper, seeded and diced
- ✓ 1 green pepper, seeded and diced

Directions:

- ❖ Preheat the oven to 375 degrees F. Lightly grease a large baking tray.
- ❖ In a large bowl, add all the ingredients and mix well.

Ingredients:

- ✓ 1 onion, thinly sliced
- ✓ 1 tablespoon pure maple syrup
- ✓ 2 tablespoons of olive oil
- ✓ Sea salt and freshly ground black pepper, to taste

- ❖ Transfer the vegetable mixture into the prepared baking tin.
- ❖ Bake for about 15-20 minutes.
- ❖ Remove from the oven and serve immediately.

81) Vegetarian Ratatouille

Preparation time: 20 minutes   **Cooking time:** 45 minutes   **Portions: 4**

Ingredients:

- ✓ 6 ounces of homemade tomato paste
- ✓ 3 tablespoons of olive oil, divided by
- ✓ ½ onion, chopped
- ✓ 3 tablespoons minced garlic
- ✓ Sea salt and freshly ground black pepper, to taste
- ✓ 1 courgette, cut into thin circles

Directions:

- ❖ Preheat the oven to 375 degrees F.
- ❖ In a bowl, add the tomato paste, 1 tablespoon of oil, onion, garlic, salt and black pepper and mix well.
- ❖ On the bottom of a 10x10 inch baking tray, spread the tomato paste mixture evenly.
- ❖ Arrange the vegetable slices alternately, starting at the outer edge of the pan and working concentrically towards the centre.

Ingredients:

- ✓ 1 yellow pumpkin, cut into thin circles
- ✓ 1 aubergine, cut into thin circles
- ✓ 1 red pepper, seeded and cut into thin rounds
- ✓ 1 yellow pepper, seeded and cut into thin rounds
- ✓ 1 tablespoon fresh thyme leaves, chopped
- ✓ 1 tablespoon fresh lemon juice
- ❖ Drizzle the vegetables with the remaining oil and sprinkle with salt and black pepper, followed by thyme.
- ❖ Place a piece of parchment paper on top of the vegetables.
- ❖ Bake for about 45 minutes.
- ❖ Remove from the oven and serve hot.

82) Quinoa with vegetables

Preparation time: 15 minutes   **Cooking time:** 26 minutes   **Portions: 4**

Ingredients:

For roasted mushrooms:
- ✓ 2 cups of small fresh Baby Bella mushrooms
- ✓ 1 tablespoon olive oil
- ✓ Sea salt, to taste

For the quinoa:
- ✓ 2 cups of alkaline water
- ✓ 1 cup of red quinoa, rinsed
- ✓ 2 tablespoons fresh parsley, chopped

Directions:

- ❖ Preheat the oven to 425 degrees F. Line a large rimmed baking sheet with baking paper.
- ❖ In a bowl, add the mushrooms, oil and salt and stir to coat well.
- ❖ Arrange the mushrooms on the prepared baking tray in a single layer.
- ❖ Roast for about 15-18 minutes, tossing once halfway through cooking.
- ❖ Meanwhile, for the quinoa: in a pan, add the water and quinoa over medium-high heat and bring to the boil.
- ❖ Reduce the heat to low and simmer, covered, for about 15-20 minutes or until all the liquid is absorbed.
- ❖ Remove from the heat and set the pan aside, covered, for about 5 minutes.
- ❖ Uncover the pan and use a fork to stir in the quinoa.

Ingredients:

- ✓ 1 clove of garlic, minced
- ✓ 1 tablespoon olive oil
- ✓ 2 teaspoons of fresh lemon juice
- ✓ Sea salt and freshly ground black pepper, to taste

For the broccoli:
- ✓ 1 cup of broccoli florets
- ✓ 2 tablespoons of olive oil

- ❖ Mix the parsley, garlic, oil, lemon juice, salt and black pepper and set aside to cool completely.
- ❖ Meanwhile, for the broccoli: in a pot of water, place a steamer basket and bring to the boil.
- ❖ Place the broccoli florets in the basket of the steamer and steam, covered, for about 5-6 minutes.
- ❖ Drain the broccoli florets well.
- ❖ Transfer the broccoli florets to the bowl with the quinoa and mushrooms and stir to combine.
- ❖ Drizzle with oil and serve immediately.

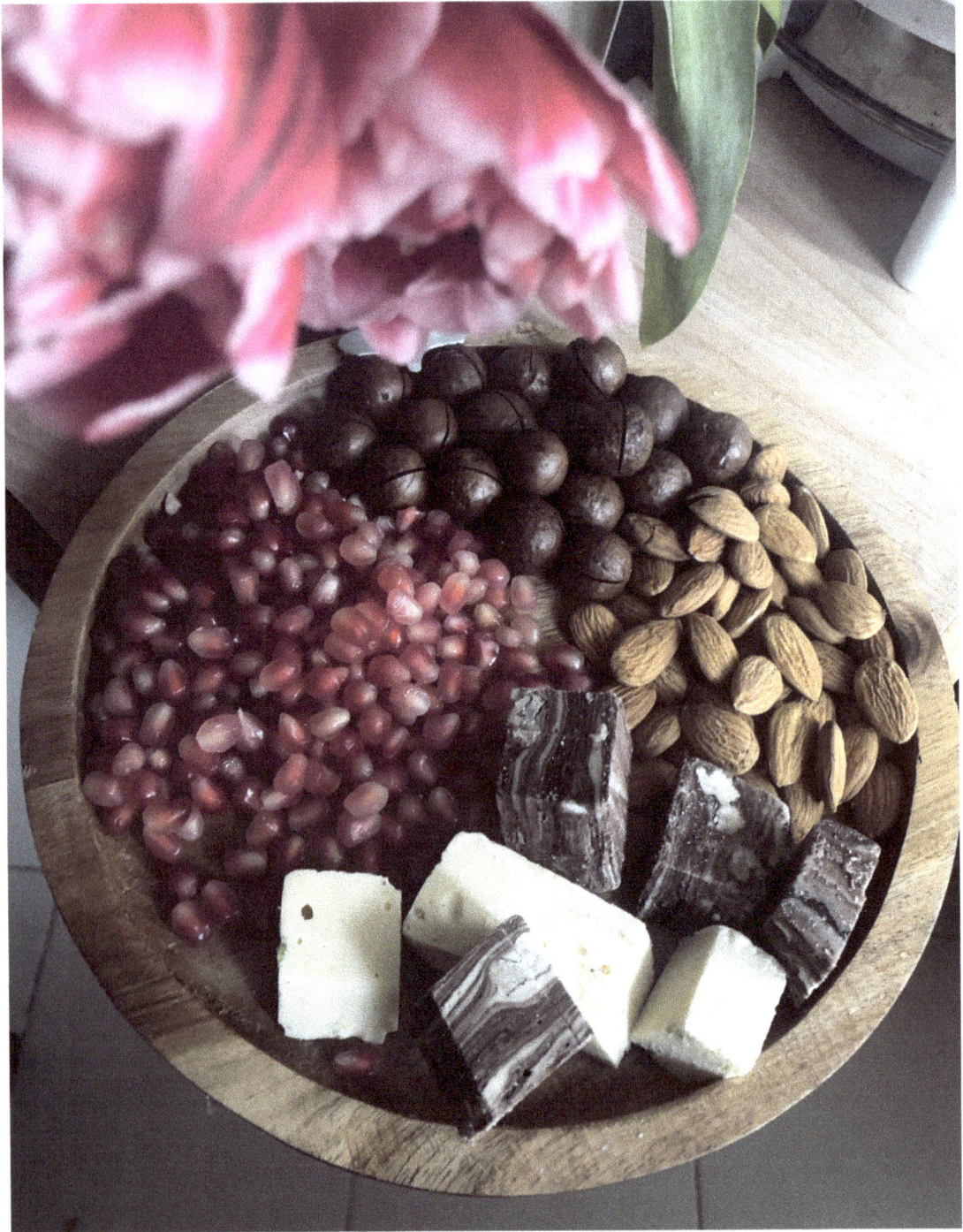

83) Bean burgers

Preparation time: 20 minutes   **Cooking time:** 25 minutes   **Portions: 8**

Ingredients:

- ½ cup walnuts
- 1 carrot, peeled and chopped
- 1 celery stalk, chopped
- 4 shallots, chopped
- 5 cloves of garlic, minced

Directions:

- ❖ Preheat the oven to 400 degrees F. Line a baking tray with baking paper.
- ❖ In a food processor, add the walnuts and pulse until finely ground.
- ❖ Add the carrot, celery, shallot and garlic and pass through a meat grinder until finely chopped.
- ❖ Transfer the vegetable mixture into a large bowl.
- ❖ In the same food processor, add the beans and give a pulse until they are chopped.

Ingredients:

- 2¼ cups canned black beans, rinsed and drained
- 2½ cups sweet potato, peeled and grated
- ½ teaspoon red pepper flakes, crushed
- ¼ teaspoon cayenne pepper
- Sea salt and freshly ground black pepper, to taste
- ❖ Add 1 1/2 cups of sweet potatoes and pulse to form a chunky mixture.
- ❖ Transfer the bean mixture to the bowl with the vegetable mixture.
- ❖ Stir in the remaining sweet potato and spices and mix until well combined.
- ❖ Make 8 patties of equal size from the dough.
- ❖ Arrange the meatballs on the prepared baking tray in a single layer.
- ❖ Bake for about 25 minutes.
- ❖ Serve hot.

84) Grilled watermelon

Preparation time: 10 minutes   **Cooking time:** 4 minutes   **Portions: 4**

Ingredients:

- 1 watermelon, peeled and cut into 1-inch-thick segments
- 1 clove of garlic, finely chopped
- 2 tablespoons fresh lime juice

Directions:

- ❖ Preheat the grill to high heat. Grease the grill grate.
- ❖ Grill the watermelon pieces for about 2 minutes on both sides.

Ingredients:

- Pinch of cayenne pepper
- Pinch of sea salt

- ❖ Meanwhile, in a small bowl, mix together the remaining ingredients.
- ❖ Sprinkle the watermelon slices with the lemon mixture and serve.

85) Mango sauce

Preparation time: 15 minutes   **Cooking time:**   **Portions: 6**

Ingredients:

- 1 avocado, peeled, pitted and diced
- 2 tablespoons fresh lime juice
- 1 mango, peeled, pitted and diced
- 1 cup cherry tomatoes, halved

Directions:

- ❖ In a large bowl, add the avocado and lime juice and mix well.

Ingredients:

- 1 jalapeño pepper, seeded and chopped
- 1 tablespoon fresh coriander, chopped
- Sea salt, to taste

- ❖ Add the remaining ingredients and stir to combine.
- ❖ Serve immediately.

86) Avocado gazpacho

Preparation time: 15 minutes   **Cooking time:**   **Portions: 6**

Ingredients:

- 3 large avocados, peeled, pitted and chopped
- 1/3 cup fresh coriander leaves
- 3 cups of homemade vegetable stock
- 2 tablespoons fresh lemon juice

Directions:

- ❖ Add all ingredients to a high-speed blender and pulse until smooth.

Ingredients:

- 1 teaspoon ground cumin
- ¼ teaspoon cayenne pepper
- Sea salt, to taste

- ❖ Transfer the soup into a large bowl.
- ❖ Cover the bowl and refrigerate for at least 2-3 hours before serving.

87) Roasted chickpeas

Preparation time: 10 minutes   **Cooking time:** 45 minutes   **Portions: 12**

Ingredients:

- ✓ 4 cups of cooked chickpeas
- ✓ 2 cloves of garlic, minced
- ✓ ½ teaspoon dried oregano, crushed
- ✓ ½ teaspoon of smoked paprika

Ingredients:

- ✓ ¼ teaspoon of ground cumin
- ✓ Sea salt, to taste
- ✓ 1 tablespoon olive oil

Directions:

- ❖ Preheat the oven to 400 degrees F. Grease a large baking tray.
- ❖ Arrange the chickpeas on the prepared baking tray in a single layer.
- ❖ Roast for about 30 minutes, stirring the chickpeas every 10 minutes.
- ❖ Meanwhile, in a small bowl, mix together the garlic, thyme and spices.
- ❖ Remove the baking tray from the oven.
- ❖ Pour the garlic and oil mixture over the chickpeas and stir to coat them well.
- ❖ Roast for another 10-15 minutes or so.
- ❖ Now, turn off the oven but leave the pan for about 10 minutes before serving.

88) Banana chips

Preparation time: 10 minutes   **Cooking time:** 1 hour and 10 minutes   **Portions:**

Ingredients:

- ✓ 2 large bananas, peeled and cut into ¼ inch thick slices

Ingredients:

Directions:

- ❖ Prepare the oven for 250 degrees F. Line a large baking tray with baking paper.
- ❖ Arrange the banana slices on the prepared baking tray in a single layer.
- ❖ Bake for about 1 hour.

89) Roasted cashews

Preparation time: 10 minutes   **Cooking time:** 10 minutes   **Portions: 12**

Ingredients:

- ✓ 2 cups of raw cashews
- ✓ ½ teaspoon ground cumin
- ✓ ¼ teaspoon cayenne pepper

Ingredients:

- ✓ Pinch of salt
- ✓ 1 tablespoon fresh lemon juice

Directions:

- ❖ Preheat the oven to 400 degrees F. Line a large baking tray with a piece of foil.
- ❖ In a large bowl, add the cashews and spices and stir to coat well.
- ❖ Transfer the cashews to the prepared baking tray.
- ❖ Roast for about 8-10 minutes.
- ❖ Sprinkle with lemon juice and serve.

90) Dried orange slices

Preparation time: 10 minutes   **Cooking time:** 1 hour   **Portions: 15**

Ingredients:

- ✓ 4 seedless navel oranges, thinly sliced (DO NOT peel the oranges)

Ingredients:

Directions:

- ❖ Set the dehydrator to 135 degrees F.
- ❖ Place the orange slices on the sheets of the dehydrator.
- ❖ Dehydrate for about 10 hours.

91) Chickpea hummus

Preparation time: 10 minutes   **Cooking time**:   **Portions: 12**

Ingredients:

- ✓ 2 (15-ounce) cans of chickpeas, rinsed and drained
- ✓ ½ cup of tahini
- ✓ 1 clove of garlic, chopped
- ✓ 2 tablespoons fresh lemon juice

Directions:

- ❖ In a blender, add all the ingredients and pulse until smooth.

Ingredients:

- ✓ Sea salt, to taste
- ✓ Filtered water, if necessary
- ✓ 1 tablespoon olive oil plus more for spraying
- ✓ Pinch of cayenne pepper
- ❖ Transfer the hummus to a large bowl and drizzle with oil.
- ❖ Sprinkle with cayenne pepper and serve immediately.

92) Avocado fries in the oven

Preparation time: 7 minutes   **Cooking time**: 17 minutes   **Portions: 4**

Ingredients:

- ✓ ½ cup of almond flour
- ✓ ½ teaspoon ground paprika, plus more for sprinkling
- ✓ 2 tablespoons nutritional yeast
- ✓ ½ teaspoon of garlic powder

Directions:

- ❖ Preheat the oven to 420°F.
- ❖ In a small bowl, mix together the almond flour, nutritional yeast, garlic powder, paprika and salt until well combined.
- ❖ Halve and pit the avocados, and split each half from pole to pole. Remove the skin.
- ❖ Add the almond milk in another small bowl.
- ❖ Line a baking tray with baking paper.

Ingredients:

- ✓ 2 avocados, slightly unripe
- ✓ ½ cup of almond milk
- ✓ ½ teaspoon of sea salt

- ❖ Dip one avocado slice first in the milk and then in the coating mixture, turning it gently to make sure it is completely covered, and place it on the prepared baking tray. Repeat with the other avocado slices.
- ❖ Bake for 15-17 minutes, taking care not to overcook or burn them.
- ❖ Remove from the oven, sprinkle with more paprika and serve immediately.

93) Dried apples with cinnamon

Preparation time: 3 minutes   **Cooking time**: 3 hours   **Portions: 1**

Ingredients:

- ✓ 2 apples, sliced
- ✓ 1 teaspoon ground cinnamon

Directions:

- ❖ Spread all the apple slices on a baking tray.
- ❖ Cough up the slices with cinnamon and olive oil.

Ingredients:

- ✓ 1 teaspoon of olive oil

- ❖ Bake for 3 hours at 200 degrees F.
- ❖ Serve and enjoy!

94) Guacamole sauce

Preparation time: 5 minutes   **Cooking time**:   **Portions: 1**

Ingredients:

- ✓ ½ cup of sauce,
- ✓ 2 crushed avocados,

Directions:

- ❖ Mix all ingredients in a bowl.

Ingredients:

- ✓ 2 tablespoons chopped coriander
- ✓ Salt, to taste

- ❖ Serve and enjoy!

95) Apple chips

Preparation time: 3 minutes

Cooking time: 40 minutes

Portions: 2

Ingredients:

- ✓ 2 apples, core and thin slices
- ✓ 2 tablespoons of white sugar

Ingredients:

- ✓ ½ teaspoon ground cinnamon

Directions:

- ❖ Preheat the oven to 225 degrees F.
- ❖ Place the apple slices on a baking tray.

- ❖ Sprinkle with cinnamon and sugar.
- ❖ Bake for 40 minutes and then serve.

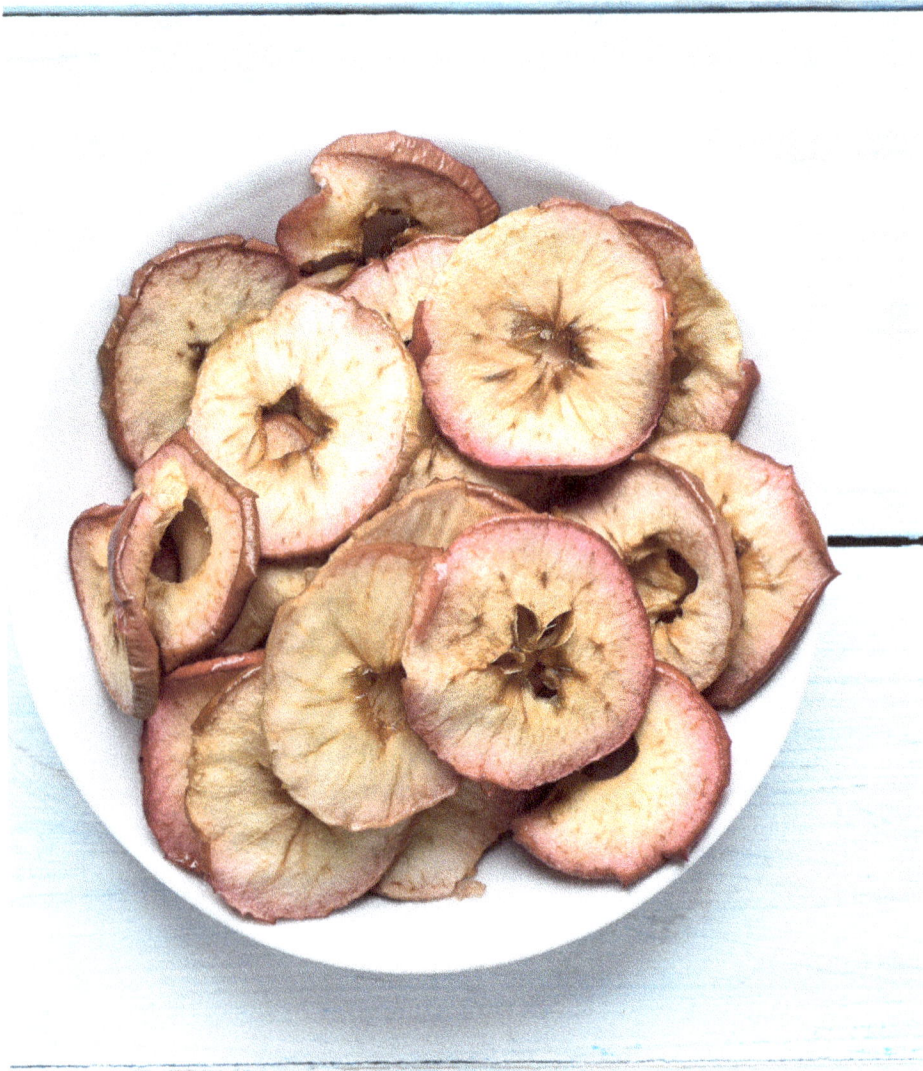

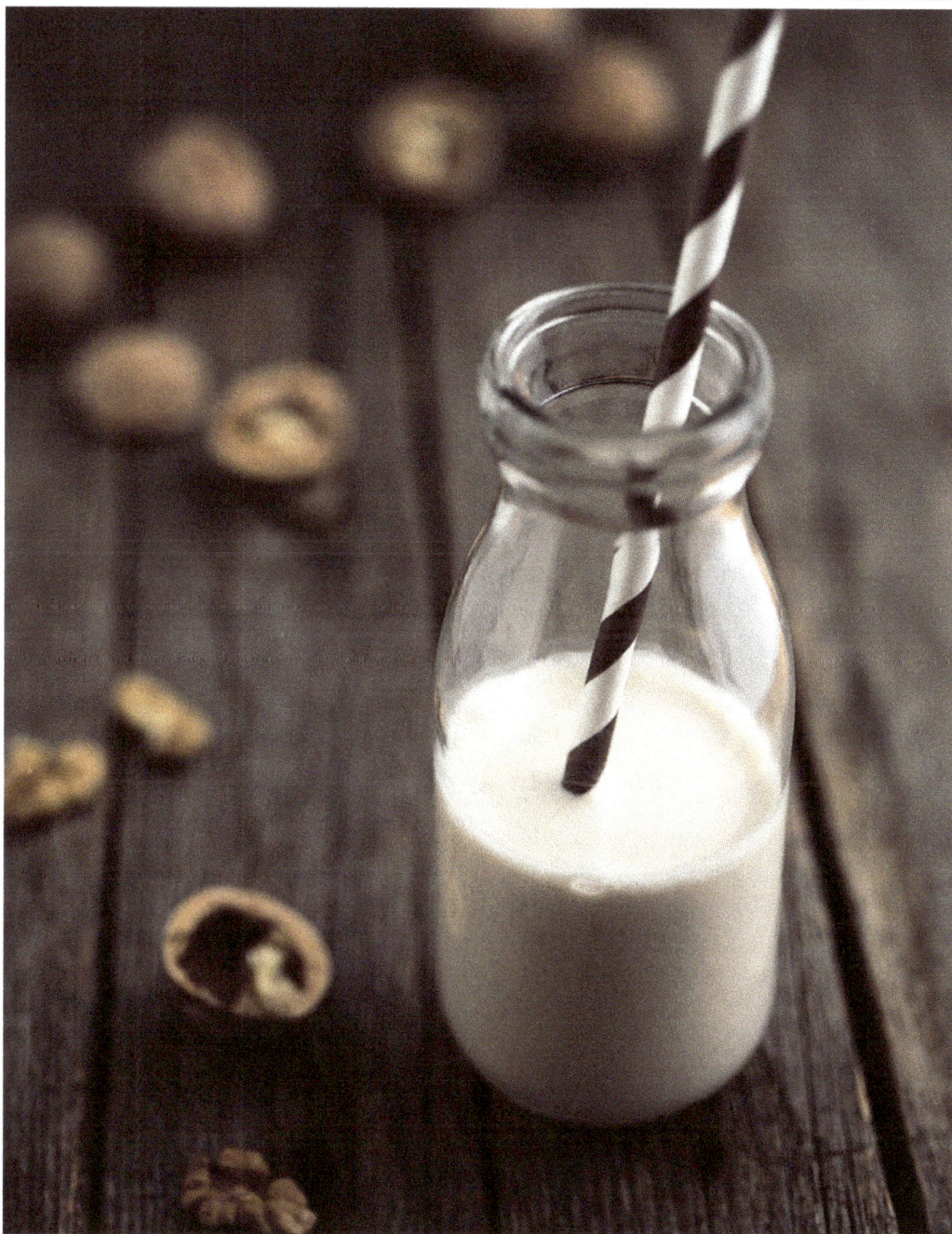

96) Strawberry Sorbet

Preparation time: 4 hours **Cooking time**: **Portions: 4**

Ingredients:
- ✓ 2 cups of Strawberries*.
- ✓ 1 1/2 teaspoons of spelt flour

Directions:
- ❖ Add the Date sugar, water and Spelt flour to a saucepan and simmer for about ten minutes. The mixture should look like a syrup.
- ❖ Remove the meat from the cap and let it rest.
- ❖ After cooling, add the Strawberry puree and stir.
- ❖ Put this mixture in a container and freeze.

Ingredients:
- ✓ 1/2 cup Date sugar
- ✓ 2 cups of Spring Water

- ❖ Cut it into pieces, put the butter in a bowl and beat until it reaches the limit.
- ❖ Put all the butter in the container and leave it in a cool place for at least four hours.
- ❖ Serve and enjoyy your Strawberry Sorbet!

Helpful hints: If you don't have fresh berries, you can use frozen ones.

97) Blueberry muffins

Preparation time: 1 hour **Cooking time**: **Portions: 3**

Ingredients:
- ✓ 1/2 cup of Blueberries
- ✓ 3/4 cup of Teff Flour
- ✓ 3/4 cup of Spelt Flour
- ✓ 1/3 cup of Agave Syrup

Directions:
- ❖ Preheat our oven to 365 degrees Fahrenheit.
- ❖ Grate or line up 6 standard muffin cups.
- ❖ Add the yeast, sifted flour, mashed potato, nut milk, peanut butter and agave juice to a large bowl.

Ingredients:
- ✓ 1/2 teaspoon of Pure Sea Salt
- ✓ 1 cup of Coconut Milk
- ✓ 1/4 cup of Sea Moss Gel seed oil (optional, check information)

- ❖ Put them in order for a while.
- ❖ Add the blueberries to the mixture and mix well.
- ❖ Divide muffin batter among 6 muffin cups.
- ❖ Bake for 30 minutes until golden brown.
- ❖ Serve and enjoy your Blueberry Muffins!

98) Banana Strawberry Ice Crem

Preparation time: **Cooking time**: 4 Hours **Portions: 5**

Ingredients:
- ✓ 1 cup of Strawberry*.
- ✓ 5 quartered Baby Bananas*.
- ✓ 1/2 Avocado, chopped

Directions:
- ❖ Put all the ingredients together and let them dry well.
- ❖ Taste. If so, add more milk or agave syrup if you want it to be more full-bodied.

Ingredients:
- ✓ 1 tablespoon of Agave syrup
- ✓ 1/4 cup of nut milk Homemade

- ❖ Place in a container with a lid and leave to mash for at least 5-6 hours.
- ❖ Serve and enjoy your Bana Strawberry Ice creamy!

Helpful hints: If you don't fresh berries or banas, you can use frozen ones. You can use as much fruit as you want, but make sure you use only fresh fruit. The fat in the Avocado helps make a creamier consissitency. If you don't have homemade nut milk, you can replace it with homemade sheep's milk.

99) Chocolate cream Homemade Whipped

Preparation time: 10 Minutes.   **Cooking time**:   **Servings: 1 cup**

Ingredients:

✓   1 cup of Aquafaba

Directions:

❖   Add Agave Syrup and Aquafaba into a bowl.
❖   Mix to the height speed about 5 minutes with a mixer support o 10 to 15 minutes with a mixer hand.

Ingredients:

✓   1/4 cup of Agave Syrup
❖   Serve and enjoy our Homemade Whipped Cream!

Helpful hints: Keep in the refrigerator if not using immediately. The whipped cream will become Aquafaba consistency eventually, until set.

100)   "'Chocolate' Pudding.

Preparation time: **Cooking time**: 20 Minutes.   **Portions: 4**

Ingredients:

✓   1 to 2 cups of Black Sapote
✓   1/4 cup agave syrup
✓   1/2 cup of soaked Brazil Nuts (overnight or at least 3 hours)

Directions:

❖   Cut 1 or 2 cups of Black Sapote in half.
❖   Remove all seeds. You should have 1 cup ou full of fruit de-seded.

Ingredients:

✓   1 tablespoon hemp seeds
✓   1/2 cup of Spring Water

❖   Place all the ingredients in a blender and blend until smooth.
❖   Serve and enjoy our chocolate pudding!

Helpful hints: Store in the fridge if not in use. You can use it with our Homemade whipped crust.

101)   Walnut muffins

Preparation time: **Cooking time**: 1 hour   **Portions: 6**

Ingredients:

✓   Dry ingredients:
✓   1 1/2 cups of Spell or Teff Flour
✓   1/2 teaspoon of Pure Sea Salt
✓   3/4 cup of Date Syrup
✓   What is the problem?
✓   2 medium pureed Burro Banas

Directions:

❖   Preheat the oven to 400 degrees.
❖   Take a muffin tray and grease 12 cups or line with cupcake liners.
❖   Place all the dry ingredients in a large bowl and mix well.
❖   Add all the ingredients to a larger bowl and mix with the Bin Laden. 5. Mix the ingredients from the two bowls into one container. Be careful not to overmix.

Ingredients:

✓   ¼ cup of ground soya oil
✓   ¾ cup of Homemade Walnut Milk *
✓   1 tablespoon Key Lime Juice
✓   Ingredients for filling:
✓   ½ cup of chopped Walnuts (plus extra for decorating)
✓   1 banana burrita
❖   Add the filling ingredients and fry.
❖   Place our batter in the 12 muffin cases and fill them with a knob of butter.
❖   Bake 22 to 26 mnutes until golden brown.
❖   Allow to cool for 10 minutes.
❖   Serve and enjoy your Bana Nut Muffins!

Useful tips:

102) Walnut cheesecake Mango

Preparation time: **Cooking time:** 4 hours 30 minutes   **Portions:** 8

Ingredients:
- ✓ 2 cups of Brazil Nuts
- ✓ 5 to 6 Dates
- ✓ 1 tablespoon of Sea Moss Gel (check information)
- ✓ 1/4 cup o agave syrup
- ✓ 1/4 teaspoon salt Pure Sea
- ✓ 2 tbsp. of Lime Juice
- ✓ 1 1/2 cups of Homemade Walnut Milk *

Directions:
- ❖ Put all crust ingredients in a processor and blend for 30 seconds.
- ❖ Prepare a baking tray with a sheet of parchment and roll out the loose dough with butter.
- ❖ Put the Mango sliced across the crust and freeze for 10 minutes.
- ❖ Place all the glass pieces in a bowl until ready.

Ingredients:
Crust:
- ✓ 1 1/2 cups of quartered Dates 1/4 cup of Agave Syrup
- ✓ 1 1/2 cups of Coconut Flakes
- ✓ 1/4 teaspoon of Pure Sea Salt
- ✓ Toppings:
- ✓ Mango of Sliced
- ✓ Sliced strawberries
- ❖ Place the filling on top of the butter, wrap it in aluminium foil or a food container and leave it to rest for 3 to 4 hours in the fridge.
- ❖ Take out dalla baking form and garnish with toppings.
- ❖ Serve and enjoy our Mango Nut Cheesecake!

Helpful hints: If you do not have homemade nut milk, you can use Homemade hemp seed milk.

103) Blackberry Jam

Preparation time: **Cooking time:** 4 hours 30 minutes   **Servings: 1 cup**

Ingredients:
- ✓ 3/4 cup of Blackberries
- ✓ 1 tablespoon lime juice Key

Directions:
- ❖ Place the blackberries in a medium saucepan and cook over a low heat.
- ❖ Stir in the blackberries until the liquid has disappeared.
- ❖ Once the berries have been picked, use your blender to chop up the larger pieces. If you don't have a blender, put the mixture in an immersion blender, mix it well and then put it back in the oven.

Ingredients:
- ✓ 3 tablespoons of Agave Syrup
- ✓ ¼ cup of Sea Moss Gel + extra 2 tablespoons (check information)
- ❖ Add Sea Moss Gel, Key Lime Juice and Agave Syrup to the mixture. Cook over low heat and stir well until dry.
- ❖ Remove from the heat and let it rest for 10 minutes.
- ❖ Serve with pieces or flat bread.
- ❖ Enjoy your jam!

Helpful hints: If you don't have Sea Moss Gel, you can omit it. However, the gel gives your skin a thinner, longer-lasting look. Blackberries have a natural pectin, which can have a similar effect. Store this Blackberry Jam in a glass jar with a lid in the refrigerator for 2 to 3 weeks. Do not store at extreme temperatures!

104) Blackberry Bars

Preparation time: **Cooking time:** 1 hr 20 Minutes   **Portions: 4**

Ingredients:
- ✓ 3 Burro Banas or 4 Baby Banas
- ✓ 1 cup of Spelt Flour
- ✓ 2 cups of Quinoa Flakes
- ✓ 1/4 cup of Agave Syrup

Directions:
- ❖ Set the oven to 350 degrees Fahrenheit.
- ❖ Mash the bananas with a fork in a large bowl.
- ❖ Add Agave Syrup and Grape Seed Oil to the puree and mix well.
- ❖ Add the Spelt flour and Quinoa flakes. Knead the dough until it becomes sticky to the finger.
- ❖ Prepare a 9x9-inch basket with a parchment lid.
- ❖ Take 2/3 of the dough and roll it out with your fingers on the baking tray parchment pan.

Ingredients:
- ✓ 1/4 teaspoon of Pure Sea Salt
- ✓ 1/2 cup of Grape Seed Oil
- ✓ 1 cup of prepared Blackberry Jam

- ❖ Spread Blackberry Jam over the dough.
- ❖ Crumble the rice and put it on the plate.
- ❖ Bake for 20 minutes.
- ❖ Remove from the oven and leave to cool for 10-15 minutes.
- ❖ Cut into small pieces.
- ❖ Try and enjoy our Blackberry Bars!

Helpful hints: You can store this Blackberry Bar in the fridge for 5-6 days or in the freezer for up to 3 months.

105) Squash Pie.

Preparation time:

Cooking time: 2 hours 30 Minutes   **Portions: 6-8**

Ingredients:

- ✓   2 Butternut Squashes
- ✓   1 1/4 cups of spelt flour
- ✓   1/4 cup dry sugar
- ✓   1/4 cup of Agave Syrup
- ✓   1 teaspoon of Allspice.

Ingredients:

- ✓   1 teaspoon of Pure Sea Salt
- ✓   1/4 cup soya water
- ✓   1/3 cup of fatty seed oil
- ✓   1/4 cup hemp seed milk Homemade *

Directions:

- ❖   Rinse and peel butternut pumpkins.
- ❖   Cut them in half and use a spoon to de-sed.
- ❖   Cut the meat into one piece and place it in a glass container.
- ❖   Cover the squash in Spring Water and boilte for 20-25 minutes until coooked.
- ❖   Turn off the oven and mash the cooked pumpkin.
- ❖   Add the date sugar, agave syrup, 1/8 pure sea salt and homemade milk and mix everything together.
- ❖   Crust:
- ❖   Preheat the oven to 350 degrees Fahrenheit.
- ❖   In a bowl, add the spelt flour, 1/2 teaspoon of Pure Sea Salt, Spring Water, and Grape Sed Oil and mix.

- ❖   Reduce the rice into a loaf. Add more water or flour if necessary. Leave to rest for 5 minutes.
- ❖   Spread out Spelt Flour on a piece of parchment paper.
- ❖   Roll out on a rolling pin, adding more flour to prevent sticking.
- ❖   Place the mixture in a cake tin and bake in the oven for 10 minutes.
- ❖   Remove the butter from the oven, add the filling and bake for a further 40 minutes.
- ❖   Remove the cake and leave it to stand for 30 minutes until cool.
- ❖   Serve enjoy your Squash Pie!

Useful tips:

106) Homemade Walnut Milk

Preparation time:

Cooking time: minimum 8 hours   **Servings: 4 cups**

Ingredients:

- ✓   1 cup fresh walnuts
- ✓   1/8 teaspoon of Pure Sea Salt

Ingredients:

- ✓   3 cups of spring water + extra for soaking

Directions:

- ❖   Put the new Walnuts in a bag and fill it with three tablespoons of water.
- ❖   Take the Walnuts for an hour and a half.
- ❖   Drain and rinse the nuts with warm water.

- ❖   Add the soaked walnuts, the puree and three times the spring water in a blender.
- ❖   Mix well till smooth.
- ❖   Extend it if you need to.
- ❖   Enjoy your homemade nut milk!

Useful tips:

107) Aquafaba

Preparation time:

Cooking time: 2 Hours 30 minutes   **Servings: 2-4 cups**

Ingredients:

- ✓   1 bag Garbanzo beans
- ✓   1 teaspoon of Pure Sea Salt

Ingredients:

- ✓   6 cups of Spring Water + extra for soaking

Directions:

- ❖   Put the chickpeas in a large pot, add the soy water and pure sea salt. Bring to the boil.
- ❖   Remove from the heat and leave to soak for 30 to 40 minutes.
- ❖   Filter the Garbanzo Beans and add 6 cups of water.
- ❖   Boil for 1 hr 30 minutes on medium hat.

- ❖   Filter the Garbanzo grains. This filtered water is Aquafaba.
- ❖   Pour the Aquafaba into a glass jar with a lid and place it in the refrigerator.
- ❖   After cooling, the Aquafaba becomes denser. If it is too thick, boil it for 10-20 mnutes.

Useful hints: Aquafaba is a good alternative for one egg: 2 tablespoons of Aquafaba = 1 egg white; 3 tablespoons of Aquafaba = 1 egg.

AUTHOR BIBLIOGRAPHY

THE ESSENCIAL ALKALINE DIET COOKBOOK FOR BEGINNERS

100+ Alkaline Recipes to Bring Your Body Back to Balance! Healthy Recipes to Enjoy Favorite Foods for Weight-Loss!

THE ALKAINE HEALTHY DIET FOR WOMEN

The Effective Way to Follow an Alkaline Diet comprising Plant-Based Diet Recipes: Natural Ways To Prevent Diabetes! 100+ Recipes Included!

THE ALKAINE HEALTHY DIET FOR MEN

100+ Recipes to Understand pH, Eat Well, and Reclaim Your Health! Plant-Based Recipes Are Included! Boost your Weight-Loss!

THE ALKAINE HEALTHY DIET FOR KIDS

100+ Recipes for Your Health, To Lose Weight Naturally and Bring Your Body Back To Balance

THE ALKAINE FIET COOKBOOK FOR ONE

100+ Recipes to Lose Weight and Get the Benefits of an Alkaline Diet - Alkaline Smoothies Included for Your Way to Vibrant Health - Massive Energy and Natural Weight Loss! Plant-Based Recipes Are Included!

THE ALKAINE DIET FOR WOMEN AFTER 50

2 Books in 1: The Complete Alkaline Diet Guidebook for Beginners: Understand pH, Eat Well with Easy Alkaline Diet Cookbook and more than 200+ Delicious Recipes (Lose weight, Beginners, Foods & Diet, Reset Cleanse)

THE SPECIAL ALKALINE DIET FOR TWO

2 Books in 1: Guidebook for Beginners: Understand pH, Eat Well with Easy Alkaline Diet Cookbook and more than 200 Delicious Recipes! Plant-Based Recipes Are Included!

THE ALKALINE DIET FOR DADDY AND SON

2 Books in 1: For Beginners: The Ultimate Guide of Alkaline Herbal Medicine for permanent weight loss, Understand pH with 200+ Anti Inflammatory Recipes Cookbook! Plant-Based Recipes Are Included!

THE ALKALINE DIET FAST & EASY

2 Books in 1: The Complete and Exhaustive Beginner's Guide to lose Weight, Fasting and Revitalize Your Body with Plant-Based Diet including 200+ Healthy and Tasty Recipes!

THE ALKALINE DIET FOR MUM AND KIDDOS

2 Books in 1: The Simplest Alkaline Diet Guide for Beginners + 200 Easy Recipes: How to Cure Your Body, Lose Weight and Regain Your Life with Easy Alkaline Diet Cookbook! Plant-Based Recipes Are Included!

THE ALKALINE DIET TO LOSE WEIGHT FAST

3 Books in 1: The Revolution of Eating Habits to stay Healthy and Find the Best Shape. A complete Program with 300+ Recipes to Regain a Healthy Balance of the Body with Alkaline Foods and lose Weight Quickly.

THE ALKALINE DIET FOR A HEALTHY FAMILY

3 Books in 1: A Complete Guide for Beginners to Clean and Treat Your Body, Eat Well with More Than 300+ Easy Alkaline Recipes for Weight Loss and Fight Chronic Disease!

THE ALKALINE DIET HIGH-PROTEIN FOR SPORT PLAYERS

3 Books in 1: Diet for Beginners: Top 300+ Alkaline Recipes for Weight Loss with Plant Based Diet And 21 Secrets To Reset And Understand pH Right Now!

THE ALKALINE DIET FOR ABSOLUTE BEGINNERS

3 Books in 1: This Cookbook Includes: Alkaline Diet for Beginners + Alkaline Diet Cookbook, The Best Guidebook to Understanding pH Secrets with More Than 300+ Recipes for Weight Loss and Anti-Inflammatory Action!

THE ALKALINE DIET COMPLETE EDITION FOR EVERYBODY

4 Books in 1: The complete guide to eat well and Lose Weight while understanding pH and prevent disease to boost your everyday energy! 400+ Recipes with Plant-Based Recipes Included!

CONCLUSIONS

Congratulations! You made it to the end!

Thank you for making it to the end of the Alkaline Diet; we hope it was informative and provided all you need to reach your goals, whatever they may be.

With the information you have, you can now start a successful alkaline diet. Your body works best when it's not acidic. The alkaline diet ensures that your body functions at its best. The great thing is that all the food you can eat is tasty. With the recipes in this book, you won't have to worry about making dinner. So don't wait any longer. Start today, and you will see your body change for the better.

The purpose of this cookbook was to introduce readers to most of the insights regarding the alkaline diet in a comprehensive way. Therefore, the text of this book has been categorized into several sections, each of which discusses the basics, the details, what it has and what it doesn't, and recipes related to the alkaline diet. In addition, the recipe chapter is divided into subsections, ranging from breakfast to lunch, dinner, smoothies, snacks, and desserts. So take some time to travel the length of this book and experience the miraculous effects of an alkaline diet on your mind and health.

Laura Green

www.ingramcontent.com/pod-product-compliance
Lightning Source LLC
Chambersburg PA
CBHW080630030426
42336CB00018B/3147